Viva Questions in Obstetrics, Gynecology, Psychiatry and Pediatric Nursing

Veena Rajput MSc Nursing (Obstetrics)
Reader
HOD (Obs and Gyn)
Shri Shankaracharya College of Nursing
Bhilai, Chhattisgarh, India

Chandramani MSc Nursing (Psychiatric)
Reader
Government College of Nursing, Raipur
Chhattisgarh, India

Foreword
Archana Selvan

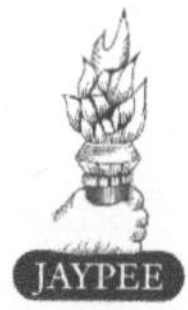

JAYPEE BROTHERS MEDICAL PUBLISHERS
The Health Sciences Publisher
New Delhi | London

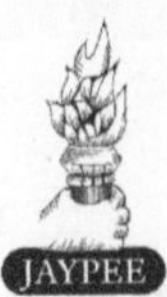

Jaypee Brothers Medical Publishers (P) Ltd

Headquarters
EMCA House
23/23-B, Ansari Road, Daryaganj
New Delhi 110 002, India
Landline: +91-11-23272143,
+91-11-23272703
+91-11-23282021, +91-11-23245672
E-mail: jaypee@jaypeebrothers.com

Corporate Office
Jaypee Brothers Medical Publishers (P) Ltd.
4838/24, Ansari Road, Daryaganj
New Delhi 110 002, India
Phone: +91-11-43574357
Fax: +91-11-43574314
E-mail: jaypee@jaypeebrothers.com

Overseas Office
JP Medical Ltd.
83, Victoria Street, London
SW1H 0HW (UK)
Phone: +44-20 3170 8910
E-mail: info@jpmedpub.com

EU GPSR Authorised Representative
Logos Europe, 9 rue Nicolas Poussin
17000, La Rochelle, France
Phone: +33 (0) 6 67 93 73 78
E-mail: Contact@logoseurope.eu

Website: www.jaypeebrothers.com
Website: www.jaypeedigital.com

© 2015, Jaypee Brothers Medical Publishers

The views and opinions expressed in this book are solely those of the original contributor(s)/author(s) and do not necessarily represent those of editor(s) of the book.

All rights reserved. No part of this publication may be reproduced, stored or transmitted in any form or by any means, electronic, mechanical, photocopying, recording or otherwise, without the prior permission in writing of the publishers.

All brand names and product names used in this book are trade names, service marks, trademarks or registered trademarks of their respective owners. The publisher is not associated with any product or vendor mentioned in this book.

Medical knowledge and practice change constantly. This book is designed to provide accurate, authoritative information about the subject matter in question. However, readers are advised to check the most current information available on procedures included and check information from the manufacturer of each product to be administered, to verify the recommended dose, formula, method and duration of administration, adverse effects and contraindications. It is the responsibility of the practitioner to take all appropriate safety precautions. Neither the publisher nor the author(s)/editor(s) assume any liability for any injury and/or damage to persons or property arising from or related to use of material in this book.

This book is sold on the understanding that the publisher is not engaged in providing professional medical services. If such advice or services are required, the services of a competent medical professional should be sought.

Every effort has been made where necessary to contact holders of copyright to obtain permission to reproduce copyright material. If any have been inadvertently overlooked, the publisher will be pleased to make the necessary arrangements at the first opportunity.

Inquiries for bulk sales may be solicited at: jaypee@jaypeebrothers.com

Viva Questions in Obstetrics, Gynecology, Psychiatry and Pediatric Nursing

First Edition: 2015, Reprint: **2025**

ISBN: 978-93-5152-677-3

Printed in India

Dedicated
to

Nursing Students
Who have Showered Love and Affection upon Us

Foreword

Practice makes perfect. I am not sure this is always the case, but practice certainly helps in knowledge acquisition and exam preparation. This book has been created by enthusiastic young teachers, who both practice and teach these specialties as part of their weekly lives.

In my opinion, the clinical specialties covered in this book are fascinating and exciting areas of the nursing curriculum.

Knowledge and understanding of these areas of clinical practice are essential and what is the better way to check your knowledge than by answering questions on the subject? This book will help and guide you. Good luck!

Dr (Prof) Archana Selvan
MSc MPhil PhD
Principal
RKDF College of Nursing
Bhopal (MP)

Preface

It gives us immense pleasure and satisfaction in introducing a guide on viva questions in nursing. The textbooks available are focused on large theoretical knowledge. This imposes students to learn vast matter on each book in nursing.

We ultimately decided to write a compact, comprehensive and practically-oriented book of nursing. This book aims at reducing the anxiety and stress during exam periods. This book will be a help to the students by providing them with instant, short and accurate answers to the questions asked during viva voce. It provides easy way to remember the points and memorize the facts in sequence without ambiguity.

The primary readers of this book will be the undergraduate students who are learning gynecology and midwifery, psychiatric and pediatric nursing, i.e. BSc Nursing 3rd and 4th year students. This book has been written in simple style and has been kept handy so that student nurses will be delighted to use it anywhere during their preparation of examination.

We hope that this guide is an earnest attempt to give enough exposure to nursing knowledge in a nutshell. We assure sure success of this guide's readers by achieving good grades in practical and competitive exams.

We are aware that for manifold reasons, errors might have crept in and shall feel obliged, if such errors are brought to our notice. These suggestions will help us to improve and bring about an improvised learning in other publication.

Veena Rajput
Chandramani

Acknowledgments

Any author, who has interest for writing any book needs help and encouragement of other persons which is very essential.

We take this opportunity to express our sincere gratitude to Prof (Mrs) Sindhu Anil Menon for being a constant guiding spirit throughout and for consistent encouragement while writing this book on nursing.

We also take this opportunity to express our sincere gratitude to Dr (Mrs) Archana Selvan who has been kind enough to go through our manuscript of this book and accepted to write FOREWORD of this book.

We are thankful to Mrs Shiny Saju for her support and Mr Nurul Hoda for typing the manuscript, our colleagues and well-wishers who have helped us in bringing out this presentation either directly or indirectly. Our heartfelt thanks to management consultant and the staff of Jaypee Brothers Medical Publishers (P) Ltd, New Delhi, India for giving a proper shape in bringing out this Viva Book in Nursing.

From the Publisher's Desk

We request all the readers to provide us their valuable suggestions/errors (if any)

at: ***jppgmee@gmail.com***

so as to help us in further improvement of this book in the subsequent edition.

Contents

Section 1: Obstetric and Gynecological Nursing

Section 2: Psychiatric Nursing

Section 3: Pediatric Nursing

Section 1

Obstetric and Gynecological Nursing

- Obstetric and Gynecological Nursing
- Antenatal Care
- Physiological Changes During Pregnancy
- Minor Ailments in Pregnancy
- Sign and Symptoms of Pregnancy
- The Fetus in Utero
- Fetal Skull
- Female Pelvis
- Antenatal Assessment of Fetal Well-being
- Normal Labor
- Normal Puerperium
- Vomiting in Pregnancy
- Ectopic Pregnancy
- Hemorrhage in Early Pregnancy
- Multiple Pregnancies
- Hypertensive Disorders in Pregnancy
- Episiotomy
- Hematological Disorders in Pregnancy Anemia in Pregnancy
- Antepartum Hemorrhage
- Cephalopelvic Disproportion
- Gestational Diabetes
- Infertility

CHAPTER 1

Obstetric and Gynecological Nursing

FILL IN THE BLANKS

1. The smallest plane of the pelvis passes through is __________ (ischial spines)
2. Pelvic axis is __________ shaped (J)
3. __________ is the area where sutures of the fetal skull meet (Fontanelle)
4. The fertilized ovum implants in the uterus on __________ day of a 28 days cycle (6–12)
5. The protein intake needs to be increased by __________ gm/day during pregnancy (15)
6. During pregnancy daily requirement of elemental iron is about __________ (20 mg)
7. Size of ovum is __________ mm (0·133)
8. The fetal liver is bypassed through __________ in fetal circulation (ductus venosus)
9. Puerperium is a period of __________ weeks after delivery.(six)
10. Vaginal discharge in puerperium is called __________. (lochia)
11. Methyl ergometrine is given intravenously with delivery of __________ of the baby (Anterior shoulder)
12. Uterine inertia is treated with an infusion of __________ (oxytocin)
13. The abdominal girth increases by about __________ cm per week beyond 30 weeks (2)
14. The abdominal girth measures at term about __________ cm (95–100)
15. Average duration of pregnancy is __________ days (280)
16. Duration of pregnancy is __________ weeks (40)
17. Fetal breathing movement is seen on USG at __________ week. (11th)
18. Placenta forms by __________ and __________ (Chorion frondosum and decidua basalis)
19. Fetal pancreas secrete insulin at __________ week. (12th)
20. Umbilical cord has __________ arteries (2)
21. Lambda in fetal skull is __________ in shape (triangular)
22. Implantation of the embryo in the fallopian tube is called __________ pregnancy (tubal ectopic)

23. Denominator in vertex presentation is __________ (occiput)
24. Medical termination of pregnancy can be done up to __________ weeks (20)
25. Occurrence of __________ or more consecutive spontaneous abortions is called habitual abortion. (3)
26. Vesicular mole may be followed by development of __________ (choriocarcinoma)
27. __________ is found in amniotic fluid in acute fetal distress (Meconium)
28. The cervix should be __________ cm dilated for forceps delivery (10)
29. Placenta is said to be retained if it is not delivered in __________ minutes after delivery of the fetus. (30)
30. __________ milk is best for a newborn baby (Breast)
31. Maternal weight should increase by at least __________ gm every week (225)
32. Maternal weight should not increase by more than __________ gm/month (2250)
33. __________ is used in the treatment of eclampsia. (Magnesium sulphate)
34. Anemia is treated with __________ and __________ (iron and folic acid)
35. Pregnancy induced hypertension is characterized by __________ and __________ (Hypertension, edema and albuminuria)
36. Fetal heart rate goes above 160 or below 120 beats per minute in cases of __________ (Fetal distress)
37. Placenta previa is associated with __________ bleeding per vaginum (painless)
38. Copper-T is a temporary form of __________ (contraception)
39. Preterm delivery occurs between __________ and __________ week (28 and 37)
40. Methyl ergometrine is given with the delivery of the __________ of the baby. (anterior shoulder)
41. Normal fetal heart rate is __________ beats per minute (120–160 beats)
42. __________ is a permanent method of male contraception (Vasectomy)
43. Foul smelling lochia is due to __________ (puerperal sepsis)
44. The cervix must be __________ cm dilated for forceps delivery (10 cm)
45. Retention of placenta is a cause of __________ (postpartum hemorrhage)
46. Tubal ectopic pregnancy ruptures in the __________ trimester (first)
47. Suboccipitobregmatic diameter measures __________ cm (14)
48. __________ is used to induce labour (Oxytocin)
49. Medical termination of pregnancy can be done up to __________ weeks (20th)
50. Puerperium is a period of __________ weeks after childbirth (6)
51. The placenta is implanted in the __________ segment in abruption placentae (upper segment)
52. Occurance of three or more consecutive abortions is called __________ (habitual abortions)
53. Postmaturity is prolongation of pregnancy more than __________ days beyond the due date (14)
54. Excessive volume of the amniotic fluid is called __________ (polyhydramnios)
55. Reduced volume of amniotic fluid is called __________ (oligohydramnios)
56. An elderly primigravida is more than __________ years old (35)

57. A woman who has delivered viable babies more than __________ times is called a grand multipara (4)
58. The condition of newborn is assessed by __________ score (apgar score)
59. The stump of the umbilical cord falls off __________ days after delivery (7 days)
60. The vaginal opening is enlarged for childbirth by the operation of __________ (episiotomy)
61. In __________ delivery, arrested fetal head can be delivered without rotating it instrumentally (Vacuum)
62. Female sterilization can be done by minilaparotomy or __________ (Laparoscopy)
63. Copper-T needs to be changed after __________ years (3)
64. Condom and diaphragm are examples of __________ contraception (Barrier contraception)
65. The period of training of a midwife is __________ months (six month)
66. Rupture of the uterus during labour is managed by __________ (casarean section)
67. Pregnancy induced hypertension may develop before __________ weeks in a case of vesicular mole (20)
68. External cephalic version is done for a fetus in __________ and __________ (Breech presentation and transverse lie)
69. A fetus in a transverse lie which cannot be turned by external cephalic version is delivered by __________ (caesarean section)
70. __________ position of the mentum is favorable for vaginal delivery in face presentation (Anterior)
71. A brow presenting fetus can deliver vaginally if it gets converted into a __________ or __________ presentation (face or vertex presentation)
72. Uterine inertia is treated with an infusion of __________ (oxytocin)
73. Constriction ring is relaxed with __________ (amylnitrite)
74. If labor is obstructed due to a contracted pelvis, the baby is delivered by __________ (caesarean section)
75. Expulsion of the fetus up to __________ weeks of pregnancy is called an abortion (22)
76. In __________ abortion the cervix is open. (inevitable)
77. Rupture of tubal ectopic pregnancy is treated surgically by __________ (salpingectomy)
78. Bleeding from the genital tract after delivery exceeding __________ ml is called postpartum hemorrhage (500)
79. Antepartum hemorrhage may be due to __________, __________ or other causes (placenta praevia, abruption placentae)
80. In multiple pregnancy, casarean section is done if the first baby is in __________ lie (transverse)
81. Postmaturity is prolongation of pregnancy more than __________ days beyond the due date (14)
82. Sacrum is made from __________ vertebrae (5)
83. Fetal skull is made from __________ bones (5)
84. The junction of two or more sutures of the skull is known as __________ (fontanelle)

85. The junction of sagittal and coronal sutures is called __________ (bregma or anterior fontanelle)
86. The largest of all the fontanelles is __________ (anterior fontanelle)
87. Bregma is fuses at age of __________ months (18)
88. Fusion of anterior fontanelle is delayed in __________ (rickets)
89. __________ is located at the junction of the sagittal and lambdoid sutures (Lambda or Posterior fontanelle)
90. Posterior fontanelle is __________ in shape (triangular)
91. Posterior fontanelle is fuses at age of __________ week (6)
92. Biparietal diameter is measures __________ cm (9.5)
93. The fertilized ovum gets implanted on the deciduas on __________ day (6–12)
94. The weight of the uterus is __________ gm at term (900 to 1000)
95. The weight of the placenta is__________ gm at term (500 to 750)
96. Fetal parts can be felt from __________ weeks (24)
97. Fetal heart sounds can be heard from __________ weeks (24)
98. __________ is a method of natural family planning method. (Rhythm method)
99. Episiotomy is made with __________ (crowning)
100. Physiological jaundice develops more than __________ hrs after birth. (48)
101. In __________ the placenta is directly anchored to the myometrium partially or completely without any intervening deciduas (placenta accrete)
102. The infant accepts an artificial nipple but refuses the mother's nipple is called __________ (nipple confusion)
103. Breast milk is sweeter due to __________ (high lactose concentration)
104. Low birth weight baby has weight less than __________ gm (2500)
105. Very low birth weight baby has weight less than __________ gm (1500)

CHAPTER 2

Antenatal Care

Q.1. What is antenatal care?

Ans. Systematic supervision (examination and advice) of a woman during pregnancy is called antenatal care.

Q.2. What are the aims of antenatal care?

Ans.
- To screen the high-risk cases.
- To prevent or to detect and treat the earliest any complication
- To ensure continued medical surveillance and prophylaxis
- To educate the mother about pregnancy to remove fear
- To discuss with couple about time, place and mode of delivery
- To motivate the couple about to need of family planning.

Q.3. Explain meaning of following terms:

Ans.
- **Gravida:** It denotes the number of pregnancies including the present one (also include number of miscarriages)
- **Para:** It denotes the number of previous pregnancies. (Not just number of children)
- **Miscarriage (abortion):** Termination of pregnancy before 20 weeks of gestation
- **Nulligravida:** Woman who has never been pregnant.

Q.4. What is the procedure at the subsequent visit?

Ans. General check-up is done at interval of 4 weeks up to 28 weeks in 8th month twice a month. There after weekly till the expected date of delivery. (Total 13 visit)

Q.5. What should be minimum visit recommended by WHO?

Ans. There should be minimum 4 visit recommended by WHO:
- 1st visit in second trimester around 16 weeks
- 2nd visit between 24–28 weeks.
- 3rd visit at 32 weeks
- 4th visit at 36 weeks.

Q.6. What are the aims of antenatal advice?

Ans.
- To explain the importance of regular check-up
- To maintain and improve health status of woman
- To improve and tone up the psychology and to remove fear about baby.

Q.7. What should be ideal diet during pregnancy?

Ans. Diet ideally during pregnancy should be light nutritious easily digestible and rich in protein, minerals and vitamins.

Q.8. Calculation of estimated date of delivery (EDD) by Naegeles rule.

Ans. Naegeles rule for calculation of EDD is add 7 days and 9 months to LMP or subtract 3 months from LMP and add 7 days, e.g. If LMP is 22nd March the EDD will be 29th December.

Q.9. When supplementary iron therapy should be started?

Ans. Iron therapy is needed for all pregnant mothers from 16th weeks onwards.

Q.10. Which live virus vaccines are contraindicated during pregnancy?

Ans. Rubella, measles, mumps, vericella, yellow fever are contraindicated during pregnancy.

Q.11. Which Immunization is must during pregnancy?

Ans. 2 dose of tetanus toxoid is must during pregnancy
First dose to be given between 16–24 weeks
Second dose to be given between 22–30 weeks.

Q.12. How much iron and folic acid required during pregnancy?

Ans. The dietary intake of both iron and folic acid is inadequate and therefore the present practice is to prescribe 100 mg of elemental iron in addition to 500 u µg or folic acid a day in empty stomach.

Q.13. Why folic acid should be continued from first trimester?

Ans. Folic acid should be continued from first trimester because folic acid reduce the risk of neural tube defect and other birth defect like cleft lip and congenital heart disease.

Calcium requirement during pregnancy is ________ mg. (1000–1500)

Q.14. What should be amount of Amniotic fluid during pregnancy?

Ans. At 12 weeks = 50 ml
At 38 weeks = 1 liter (Max)
At 40 weeks = 800 ml
At 42 weeks = 480 ml

CHAPTER

3 Physiological Changes During Pregnancy

Q.1. Weight and length of the uterus at term is: ________ and _____ cm. (900-1000 gm and 35)

Q.2. Who first described the uterine contraction?

Ans. Braxton hicks describe uterine contraction it is also known as Braxton Hicks Contraction.

Q.3. What is Braxton hicks contraction?

Ans. Braxton hicks contraction –in the very early week of pregnancy uterus undergoes spontaneous contractions that are irregular, infrequent, spasmodic and painless without any effect on dilatation of the cervix that is not recognize by mother.

Q.4. Braxton hicks contraction is not felt in ________ pregnancy. (Abdominal)

Q.5. What are the pregnancy sign?

Ans. Goodell's Sign: softening of the cervix.

Reason: fluids accumulate inside and in between the fibers vascularity is increased specially beneath the squamous epithelium of the portio vaginalis which responsible for its bluish colouration.

Hagar's sign

- Upper part of uterus is enlarged.
- Lower part of body is empty and extremely soft the cervix is comparatively firm.

Chadwick's sign or Jacquemier's: The dark purplish red discoloration and congestion of the valva and vaginal mucous membranes detected 4th and 8th week of pregnancy.

Osiander's sign: Copious nonirritating mucoid discharge appears at 6th wks and there is increased pulsation felt trough the lateral fornices at 8th weeks.

Palmer's sign: Regular and rhythmic uterine contraction can be elicited during bimanual examination as early as 4–8 wks. During contraction the uterus become firm and well define and relax it become soft and ill define. The contraction is lost for 30 second and in relaxation phase it increases, after 10th wks relaxation phase increases so much, so it is difficult to perform.

Montgomery tubercles: The nipple become large, erectile and deeply pigmented variable number of sebaceous glands (5–15) which remain invisible in the non-pregnant state. During pregnancy the areola become hypertrophied are called Montgomery's tubercles.

Linea nigra: It is a brownish black pigmented area in the midline of abdomen.
Reason: The pigmentary changes are due to melanocyte stimulating hormone from the anterior pituitary.
Striae albicans: After delivery the scar tissues contract and obliterate the capillaries and become glistening white in appearance.
Mammary murmur: A continuous hissing murmur may be audible over the tricuspid area in the left second and third intercostals spaces called the mammary murmur.
Reason: Due to increased blood flow through the internal mammary vessels.

Q.6. What should be total weight gain during pregnancy?

Ans. Total weight gain during the course of a singleton pregnancy for a healthy woman average 11Kg (24lb).

- 1 Kg in first trimester.
- 5 Kg in second and 5 kg in third trimester.

Reproductive weight gain 6 Kg as below:

- Fetus-3·3 Kg
- Placenta-0·6 Kg
- Liquor-0·8
- Uterus-0·9 Kg
- Breast-0·4 Kg

Net maternal weight gain is 6 Kg as follows

- Increase in blood volume- 1·3 Kg
- Increase in extracellular fluid-1·2 Kg
- Accumulation of fat and protein-3·5 Kg

Q.7. Why weight recording is important during pregnancy?

Ans.
- Rapid gain in weight- if more than 0·5 Kg/weeks or more than 2 Kg a month in later month may be early sign of pre-eclampsia.
- Falling weight may suggest intrauterine growth retardation.
- Ideally weight gain should depend on pre- pregnancy body mass index (BMI) level.
- For normal BMI (20–26) is 11 to 16 Kg.
- For BMI (more than 29) should not gain more than 7 Kg.
- For underweight BMI (less than 19) allowed to gain up to 18 Kg.
- During pregnancy water retained at term is about 6·5 liters

Q.8. Why pulse rate slightly increases during pregnancy?

Ans. Pulse rate slightly increases during pregnancy to meet the additional O_2 required due to increased metabolic activity during pregnancy, the increase in cardiac output is chiefly affected by increase in stroke volume and increase in pulse rate to about 15 per minute.

Q.9. Explain briefly about regional distribution of blood flow.

Ans.
- Regional distribution of blood flow is increased–
- Uterine blood flow (normal 50 ml/min) is increased by 750 ml/min near term.
- Pulmonary blood flow (normal 600 ml/min) is increased by 2500 ml/min.
- Renal blood flow (normal 800 ml) is increased by 400 ml/min.

Q.10. Heat sensation, sweating complained by pregnant woman is due to______. (increased blood flow).

Q.11. What are the Normal Hemodynamic Changes during Pregnancy?

Ans. Normal Hemodynamic Changes During Pregnancy are:

Hemodynamic Parameter	Change During Normal Pregnancy	Change During Labor and Delivery	Change During Postpartum
Blood volume	↑ 40%–50%	↑	↓ (auto diuresis)
Heart rate	↑ 10–15 beats/min	↑	↓
Cardiac output	↑ 30%–50% above baseline	↑ Additional 50%	↓
Blood pressure	↑ 10 mm Hg	↑	↓
Stroke volume	↑ First and second trimesters; ↓ third trimester	↑ (300-500 mL/ contraction)	↓
Systemic vascular resistance	↓	↑	

Q.12. Iron loss in menstrual bleeding per cycle is ________ mg (30).

Q.13. What is the reason behind increased frequency of micturation in early and late pregnancy?

Ans. **Early pregnancy:** It may be due to resulting of osmoregulation causing increased water intake and polyuria.

In late pregnancy: Due to pressure on the bladder as the presenting part descends down the pelvis. In late pregnancy bladder mucosa becomes edematous due to venous and lymphatic obstruction cause increased frequency of micturation.

Q.14. What are the functions of placenta?

Ans. **Nutrition:** Glucose, fatty acids, amino acids, electrolytes and vitamins are supplied to the fetus across the placenta by diffusion.

Respiration: Oxygen passes from the maternal blood to the fetal blood and carbon dioxide in the opposite direction across the placenta by diffusion.

Excretion: The waste products formed by fetal metabolism are excreted across the placenta to the maternal blood.

Protection: The placenta forms a barrier between the maternal blood and the fetus and thus protects it from a number of harmful substances in the maternal bloods.

Endocrine: The placenta produces a number of hormones.

Estrogen: It is produced from the 6th week of pregnancy, in large amounts from the 12th week' it is responsible for the growth of the uterus and a number of physiological changes of pregnancy.

Progesterone: It is produced initially by the corpus luteum of pregnancy and from the 12th week by the placenta. It is responsible for the physiological changes of pregnancy and preventing expulsion of the fetus.

CHAPTER

4

Minor Ailments in Pregnancy

Q.1. What is the reason of stress incontinence in late pregnancy?

Ans. Stress incontinence in late pregnancy is due to urethral sphincter weakness.

Q.2. Why heart burn or acid reflex occur during pregnancy and write its management?

Ans. Heart burn or acid reflex occur during pregnancy due to increase level of progesterone that relaxed cardiac sphincter and regurgitation gastric acid content into the oesophagus that may produce oesophagitis that causes heart burn.

- **Management of heart burn:** Lifestyle modifications may be necessary, e·g· elevating the head of the bed 6 inches, stopping smoking, sleeping on the left side, avoiding reclining for 2-3 hrs after a meal.
- **Dietary modification:** Eating less fat and more protein, avoiding chocolate and certain drinks such as coffee, citrus juices, tomato products, antacid such as ranitidine may provide relief.

Q.3. Why constipation occur during pregnancy and write the management?

Ans. Muscle tone and motility of entire gastrointestinal tract are diminished due to high progesterone level this atonicity of the gut leads to constipation.

Q.4. __________ is responsible for calcium absorption from intestine and kidneys.

(1,25 dihydroxy vitamin D3)

Q.5. Why lumber lordosis occur during pregnancy and write it's management?

Ans. Increased mobility of the pelvic joints it leads to softening of the ligaments that causes release of relaxin, this relaxin is responsible for lumber lardosis.

Management of lumber lordosis: improvement of posture, well fitted pelvic girdle belt during walking, rest in hard bed often relieve the symptoms.

Q.6. Why haemorrhoids occur during pregnancy and write its management?

Ans. Reason: Because of constipation and pressure in veins below the level of the enlarging uterus. Poor support for hemorrhoidal veins in the anorectal area and lack of valves in these vessels can lead to reversal in the direction of blood flow and stasis of blood.

Management: Women should be offered dietary advice (high fiber diet) and if symptoms remain troublesome should consider standard hemorrhoid creams.

Q.7. hcG level is in peak at about _______ weeks of gestation. (8–10 wks)

Q.8. hcG is synthesized by _______ and _______ (placenta and fetal kidney)

Q.9. Write about placenta.

Ans. The placenta (also known as afterbirth) is an organ that connects the developing fetus to the uterine wall to allow nutrient uptake, waste elimination, and gas exchange via the mother's blood supply, fight against internal infection and produce hormones to support pregnancy.

The placenta functions as a fetomaternal organ with two components: the fetal placenta (chorion frondosum) which develops from the same blastocyst that forms the fetus, and the maternal placenta (deciduas basalis), which develops from the maternal uterine tissue.

The development of the extra–embryonic membranes begin at the moment of the differentiation of the blastocyst cells into an embryoblast and a trophoblast. The embryoblast forms the later embryo and the trophoblast the components of the embryonic appendage organs. The forming of the placenta is induced by the syncythiothrophoblast of the blastocyst, which triggers the decidual reaction of the uterine wall. This change of the endometrium depends on the stimulation by the hormones released by the ovary and placenta. The differentiation of the placenta begins with the formation of lacunae in the syncythiothrophoblast that are filled with maternal blood, which stems from the spiral arteries. The fetoplacental circulation begins in the 3rd week, when the fetal vessels connect the placenta with the tissues of the embryonic body. Over the course of the pregnancy, the placenta adapts to the needs of the growing embryo.

CHAPTER

5

Sign and Symptoms of Pregnancy

Q.1. What are the symptoms of pregnancy?

Ans. In first trimester (first 12 weeks)

- Amenorrhea also known as placental sign
- Morning sickness
- Frequency of micturation
- Breast discomfort in the form of feeling of fullness.

Sign in first trimester:

- Jacquemier's sign
- Vaginal sign or osiander's sign
- Goodell's sign
- Hagar's sign
- Palmer's sign.

Second trimester:

Symptoms

- Quickening—(feeling of life) first fetal movement felt about 18–20 wks
- Progressive enlargement of lower abdomen.

Third trimester:

Symptoms

- Amenorrhea persists
- Enlargement of the abdomen
- Lightening—Sense of relief of the pressure symptoms
- Frequency of micturation
- Fetal movements are more pronounced.

Sign

- Cutaneous changes are more prominent with increased pigmentation and striae
- Uterine shape changed from cylindrical to spherical beyond 36th weeks
- Fundal height: If the head is floating it is of 32th weeks pregnancy and if the head is engaged, it is of 40th weeks pregnancy
- Braxton-hicks contraction are more evident
- Fetal movements are easily felt:
- Palpation of the fetal parts and their identification become much easier.

Q.2. First fetal movement is known as _______ (quickening)

Q.3. What is pseudocyesis?

Ans. It is a psychological disorder where the woman has false but firm belief that she is pregnant although no pregnancy exists.

CHAPTER 6

The Fetus in Utero

DEFINE THE TERMS

Lie: The lie refers to the relationship of the long axis of the fetus to the long axis of the centralized uterus or maternal spine.

Presenting Part: The presenting part is defined as the part of the presentation which overlies the internal os.

Attitude: The relation of the different parts of the fetus to one another is called attitude of the fetus.

Denominator: It is an arbitrary bony fixed point on the presenting part which comes in relation with the various quadrants of the maternal pelvis denominators are:

- Occiput in vertex
- Mentum in face
- Frontal eminence in brow
- Sacrum in breech
- Acromion in shoulder

Position: It is the relation of the denominator to the different quadrants of the pelvis.

Q.1. What are the conditions in which the height of uterus will be more than the period of amenorrhea?

Ans. The conditions are as follows:

- Mistaken date of the last menstrual period
- Twins
- Polyhydramnios
- Big baby
- Pelvic tumors-ovarian fibroid
- Hydatidiform mole
- Concealed accidental hemorrhage.

Q.2. Explain the condition where the height of the uterus is less than the period of amenorrhea.

Ans.
- Mistaken date of the last menstrual period.
- Scanty liquor amnii
- Fetal growth retardation
- Intrauterine fetal death.

Q.3. When Biparietal diameter of fetal head has passed the plane of pelvic brim is called __________. (engagement)

CHAPTER

7

Fetal Skull

Q.1. Write the anatomy of fetal skull.

Ans. The skull is formed of the face, the vault and the base. The bones that form the skull are: two frontal bones, two parietal bones, two temporal bones wings of the sphenoid and occipital bone. The bones of the face and base are heavy and fused The bones of the vault are 2 frontal, 2 parietal and occipital. The bones of the vault are not joined thus changes in the shape of the fetal head during labor can occur due to molding.

Q.2. Define bregma.

Ans. Diamond shaped area between anterior and posterior fontanelles and parietal eminences is called bregma.

Q.3. Define anterior fontanelle and when it is ossified or close?

Ans. Anterior fontanelle is diamond shaped space between coronal and sagittal suture 3 × 3 cm, ossifies at 18 months.

Q.4. Define Posterior fontanelle (lambda) and when it is ossified or close?

Ans. Posterior fontanelle is triangle shaped space between sagittal and lambdoid suture, it ossifies at 6–8 weeks.

Q.5. Anatomy of fetal skull.

Ans. Fetal skull: The skull is formed of the face, the vault and the base the bones that form the skull are: two frontal bones, two parietal bones, two temporal bones wings of the sphenoid and occipital bone the bones of the face and base are heavy and fused The bones of the vault are 2 frontal, 2 parietal and occipital. The bones of the vault are not joined thus changes in the shape of the fetal head during labor can occur due to molding.

Q.6. What is moulding of the head?

Ans. Moulding of the head occurs with descent of the fetal head into the pelvis to reduce the head circumference. Frontal bones slip under parietal bones. Parietal bones override each other and Parietal bones slip under the occipital bone.

Q.7. What is degree of moulding?

Ans.
- When suture lines are separate +1
- Suture lines meet +2
- Suture lines overlap but can be reduced by gentle digital pressure +3
- Overlap irreducible

Q.8. Write different parts of fetal skull

Ans. **Vertex:** It is a quadrangular area bounded anteriorly by the bregma and coronal sutures behind by the lambda and lambdoid sutures and laterally by lines passing through the parietal eminences

Brow: It is an area bounded on one side by the anterior fontanelle and coronal sutures and on the other side by the root of the nose and supraorbital ridges of either side.

Face: It is an area bounded on one side by root of the nose and supraorbital and on the other, by the junction of the floor of the mouth with neck.

Q.9. _______ is the area lying in front of the anterior fontanelle. (Sinciput)

Q.10. Wide gap in the suture line is called _______ (fontanelle).

Q.11. _______ is the alteration of the shape of the forecoming head while passing through the resistant birth passage during labor. (Moulding)

Q.12. Define sutures and types.

Ans. It is joining between two bones.

Types:
- Sagittal or longitudinal suture lies between two parietal bones
- Coronal sutures between parietal and frontal bones on either side
- The frontal suture lies between two frontal bones
- The lambdoid sutures-separate the occipital bone and the two parietal bones.

Q.13. What are the importance of sutures?

Ans. It permits gliding movement of one bone over the other during moulding of the head

Digital palpation of saggital suture during internal examination in labour.

CHAPTER 8

Female Pelvis

Q.1. What is female bony pelvis?

Ans. The female bony pelvis is divided into:

False pelvis: Above the pelvic brim and has no obstetric importance

True pelvis: Below the pelvic brim and related to the child-birth.

Q.2. What are the joints in pelvis?

Ans.
- Two sacroiliac joints
- Sacrococcygeal joint
- Symphysis pubis.

Q.3. What is the true pelvis?

Ans. The true pelvis: It is composed of inlet, cavity and outlet.

Q.4 What is the Pelvic Inlet (Brim)?

Ans. The Pelvic Inlet (Brim)

Boundaries

- Sacral promontory,
- Ala of the sacrum,
- Sacroiliac joints,
- Iliopectineal lines,
- Iliopectineal eminencies,
- Upper border of the superior pubic rami,
- Pubic tubercles,
- Pubic crests and
- Upper border of symphysis pubis.

Q.5. What are different conjugates in pelvis?

Ans. **Anatomical or anteroposterior diameter** (true conjugate conjugates) = 11 cm from the tip of the sacral promontory to the upper border of the symphysis pubis.

Obstetric conjugate = 10.5 cm from the tip of the sacral promontory to the most bulging point on the back of symphysis pubis which is about 1 cm below its upper border. It is the shortest anteroposterior diameter.

Diagonal conjugate = 12.5 cm

For example, 1.5 cm longer than the true conjugate. From the tip of sacral promontory to the lower border of symphysis pubis.

Q.6. What are the diameter of inlet?

Ans. **Anatomical anteroposterior diameter** (true conjugate or anatomical or anteroposterior conjugates) = 11 cm from the tip of the sacral promontory to the upper border of the symphysis pubis

Transverse dimeters: Anatomical transverse diameter = 13 cm between the farthest two points on the iliopectineal lines

It is the largest diameter in the pelvis

Oblique diameters: oblique diameter = 12 cm from the right sacroiliac joint to the left iliopectineal eminence.

Q.7. What is the pelvic cavity?

Ans. The pelvic cavity

It is a segment the boundaries of which are:

- The roof is the plane of pelvic brim
- The floor is the plane of least pelvic dimension
- Anteriorly the shorter symphysis pubis
- Posteriorly the longer sacrum.

Q.8. What is Pelvic Outlet and its diameter?

Ans. The pelvic outlet

Anatomical outlet: It is tablet or pill-shaped bounded by; the lower border of symphysis pubis, pubic arch, ischial tuberosities, sacrotuberous and sacrospinous ligaments and, tip of the coccyx

Obstetric outlet: It is a segment the boundaries of which are: the floor is the anatomical outlet, anteriorly the lower border of symphysis pubis, posteriorly the coccyx. laterally the ischial spines

Anteroposterior diameters: =11cm from the tip of the coccyx to the lower border of symphysis pubis

Obstetric anteroposterior diameter = 13 cm from the tip of the sacrum to the lower border of symphysis pubis as the coccyx moves backwards during the second stage of labour

Transverse diameters: Bituberous diameter = 11 cm between the inner aspects of the ischial tuberosities

Bispinous diameter = 10.5 cm between the tips of ischial spines

Posterior sagittal diameter: 7.5–10 cm from the tip of the sacrum to the centre of the bituberous diameter.

Q.9. What are different types of female pelvis?

Ans. Four types of female pelvis were described. Actually the majority of pelvis are of mixed types: Gynaecoid pelvis, Anthropoid pelvis, Android pelvis, Platypelloid pelvis.

Q.10. What are the features of gynecoid pelvis?

Ans. Classification of Pelvic Types

- Gynaecoid pelvis (50%):
- It is the normal female type
- Inlet is slightly transverse oval
- Sacrum is wide with average concavity and inclination

Side walls are straight with blunt ischial spines
Sacro-sciatic notch is wide
Subpubic angle is 90-100°.

Q.11. What are the features of anthropoid pelvis?

Ans. Anthropoid pelvis (25%):
- It is ape-like type
- All anteroposterior diameters are long
- All transverse diameters are short
- Sacrum is long and narrow
- Sacro-sciatic notch is wide
- Subpubic angle is narrow.

Q.12. What are the features of android pelvis?

Ans. Android pelvis (20%):
- It is a male type.
- Inlet is triangular or heart-shaped with anterior narrow apex.
- Side walls are converging (funnel pelvis) with projecting ischial spines.
- Sacro-sciatic notch is narrow.
- Subpubic angle is narrow < 90°.

Q.13. What are the features of platypelloid pelvis?

Ans. Platypelloid pelvis (5%): It is a flat female type
- All anteroposterior diameters are short
- All transverse diameters are long
- Sacro-sciatic notch is narrow
- Subpubic angle is wide.

Q.14. What are the criteria to assess adequacy of the pelvis to achieve vaginal delivery clinically favorable pelvis?

Ans. To assess Adequacy of the pelvis to achieve vaginal delivery clinically favorable pelvis should be as follows:
- Sacral promontory cannot be felt
- Ischial spines are not prominent
- Subpubic arch accept 2 fingers
- Intertuberous diameter accept 4 knuckles on pelvic exam.

Q.15. What are the different ligaments in pelvis?

Ans. Pelvic ligaments are:
- Sacrospinous ligament - lateral aspect of the sacrum to ischial spines
- Sacrotuberous ligament - lateral aspect of the sacrum to inner aspect of ischial tuberosity
- Sacroiliac ligament - medial surface of the ilium to sacrum
- Illiolumbar ligament - iliac crest to transvers lumbar vertebra.

Q.16. Which kind of problems encountered in contracted pelvis?

Ans. Problems encountered in contracted pelvis are:
- Small round pelvis, extreme flexion, excessive moulding, delay in 2nd stage, fetal distress, maternal distress, instrumental delivery, BVD is hazardous because of limited space for internal manipulations.

CHAPTER

9

Antenatal Assessment of Fetal Well-being

Q.1. When you will advise the ANC patient to hospitalized?

Ans.
- If painful uterine contractions at interval of about 10 minutes and continued for at least an hour suggestive of onset of labor.
- Sudden gush of watery fluid per vaginam-suggestive of premature rupture of the membranes.
- Active vaginal bleeding, however slight it may be.

Q.2. What is the main cause of fetal death during antepartum period

Ans.
- Chronic fetal hypoxia (IUGR)
- Maternal complication, e.g. diabetes, hypertension, infection
- Fetal congenital malformation
- Unexplained cause.

Q.3. Clinical examination advice to pregnant women in first visit

Ans.
a. Hemoglobin estimation
b. Routine examination of urine-culture
c. Serological tests for syphilis
d. ABO and Rh grouping
e. Estimation of post prandial blood glucose and glucose tolerance test
f. Tests for toxoplasmosis and antiphospholipid antibodies in case of recurrent abortion.

Q.4 Maternal serum alpha fetoprotein (MSAFP) is produced by________and________. (Yolk sac and fetal liver).

Q.5. Highest level of AFP (alpha fetoprotein) in fetal serum and amniotic fluid is reached around __________ (13 weeks)

Q.6. Prenatal genetic diagnosis can be made directly from fetal tissues obtained by _________ and _________ (amniocentesis and chorion villous sampling).

Q.7. What is cordocentesis?

Ans. A 25 gauze spinal needle 13 cm in length is inserted through the maternal abdominal and uterine wall under real time ultrasound guidance using a curvilinear probe. The needle tip punctures the umbilical vein approximately 1–2 cm from the placental insertion.

Generally 0.5 to 2 ml of fetal blood is collected. It is performed under local anaesthetic usually after 18 weeks of gestation.

Q.8. What is non-stress test?

Ans. It is a continuous electronic monitoring of the fetal heart rate along with recording of fetal movements. There is an observed association of FHR acceleration with fetal movements which indicates a healthy fetus.

Q.9. What are the common indication of antepartum fetal monitoring?

Ans. **a.** Pregnancy with obstetric complication: IUGR, multiple pregnancy, polyhydr-aminos

b. Pregnancy with medical complication: Diabetes mellitus, hypertension, renal or cardiac disease, infection.

Q.10. Enlist the biophysical tests are used during pregnancy

Ans.
- Fetal movement count.
- Cardiotocography
- Non stress test
- Fetal biophysical profile
- Contraction stress test
- Doppler ultrasound
- Vibroacoustic stimulation test.

Q.11. What is contraction stress test?

Ans. It is an invasive method to assess the fetal well-being during pregnancy when there is alteration in FHR in response to uterine contraction it suggests fetal hypoxia.

Q.12. What are the Indication of contraction stress test?

Ans. **a.** Intrauterine growth restriction

b. Postmaturity

c. Hypertensive disorders of pregnancy

d. Diabetes.

Q.13. When CST is contraindicated?

Ans.
- CST is contraindicated in following condition that are:
- Compromised fetus
- Previous history of caesarean section
- Complication likely to produce preterm labor
- Antepartum hemorrahage.

Q.14. How to assess the fetal well-being in late pregnancy?

Ans. There are mainly 3 methods to assess the fetal well-being in late pregnancy are:
- Clinical–by head to toe examination
- Biochemical- done for pulmonary maturity
- Biophysical- this test is done for screening of utero-placental insufficiency Bio-physical test are enlist earlier.

Q.15. How fetal biophysical activity change?

Ans. The fetal biophysical activities are initiated, modulated and regulated through fetal nervous system. The fetal CNS is very much sensitive to diminished oxygenation

Hypoxia → metabolic acidosis → CNS depression → changes in fetal biophysical activity.

Q.16. Respiratory distress syndrome (RDS) is caused by deficiency of ______ (pulmonary surfactant).

Q.17. What is RDS and write the causes of Respiratory distress syndrome?

Ans.
- RDS is respiratory distress syndrome. Specially found in preterm newborns. (< 37 weeks)
- The respiratory epithelial cells in the alveoli are of two Type. Type I and Type II
- RDS is caused by deficiency of pulmonary surfactant which is synthesized by the type II alveolar cells.
- Surfactant is packed in lamellar bodies→discharged in the lung alveoli→ carried in the pulmonary fluid→carried into the amniotic fluid.

Q.18. What is surfactant?

Ans. The respiratory epithelial cells in the alveoli are of two type.
Type I and type II. This type II alveolar cells synthesized surfactant these surfactant is estimated by lecithin and sphingomylin (L/S) ratio the level of surfactant indicate pulmonary maturity that is
- Amniotic fluid L/S ratio is 1 at 31–32 weeks
- Amniotic fluid L/S ratio is 2 at 35 weeks
- Amniotic fluid L/S ratio is 2 it indicates pulmonary maturity.

Q.19. What are the types of birth defects?

Ans. The birth defects may be:
- Chromosomal- numerical or structural
- Single gene disorder
- Polygenic or multifectorial
- Teratogenic disorder (drugs).

About half of chromosomal abnormalities are due to autosomal trisomy and remaining half is due to sex chromosomal abnormalities.

Q.20. Maternal serum Alfa Fetoprotein estimation is done between ________ weeks of gestation. (15–18)

Q.21. Normal value of MSAFP is ________mom. (2.5)

Q.22. Elevated level of MSAFP (Maternal serum Alfa Fetoprotein) indicated ________. (Open NTDs)

Q.23. What is triple test?

Ans. It is test of MSAFP, Hcg, UE3 is used for detection of Down syndrome. It is done between 15–18 weeks of gestation.

Q.24. What is Fetal Movement Count?

Ans. It is mothers first line screening test both for high risk and low risk patient. A healthy fetus should have minimum 10 movements in 12 hours period count should be done daily beginning at 28 weeks.

CHAPTER 10

Normal Labor

Q.1. Define normal labor.

Ans. The series of events that take place in the genital organs in an effort to expel the viable product of conception out of the womb through the vagina into the outer world is called labor.

Q.2. Normal labor is known as __________. (Eutocia)

Q.3. Abnormal labor is known as ________. (Dystocia)

Q.4. Write the stages of labor?

Ans. Conventionally, events of labor are divided into three stages:

- **First stage:** It starts from the onset of true labor pain and ends with full dilatation of the cervix. Its average duration is 12 hours in primigravidae and 6 hours in multiparae
- **Second stage:** It starts from the full dilatation of the cervix and ends with expulsion of the fetus from the birth canal. Its average duration is 2 hours in primigravidae and 30 minutes in multiparae
- **Third stage:** It begins after expulsion of the fetus and ends with expulsion of the placenta and membranes its average duration is about 15 minutes in both primigravidae and multiparae
- **Fourth stage:** It is the stage of observation for at least one hour after expulsion of the after birth.

Q.5. Enlist the criteria for normal labor.

Ans. The labor should be fulfill the following criteria:

- Spontaneous in onset at term.
- With vertex presentation.
- Without undue prolongation.
- Natural termination with minimal aids.
- Without having and complications affecting the health of mother or baby.
- Single live fetus.
- Baby weight should be 2500–3500 gm.

Q.6. What are the causes of onset of labor?

Ans. The precise mechanism of initiation of labor is still obscure. But following hypotheses is given below:

- **Uterine distension:** Stretching effect of myometrium
- **Feto-placental contribution:** Fetal hypothalamic pituitary adrenal axis prior to onset of labor → increased CRH → increased release of ACTH → Fetal adrenals → increased cortisol secretion→ accelerated production of oestrogen and prostaglandins from the placenta
- **Oestrogen:** It increases the release of oxytocin from maternal pituitary.

↓ causes

Synthesis of receptors for oxytocin in myometrium and deciduas.

↓

That increases the lysosomal disintegration in amnion cell that increased prostaglandin synthesis.

↓

It stimulates synthesis of myometrial contractile protein that is actomyosin through cAMP.

↓

That increased the excitability of myometrial cell membranes.

- Prostaglandin: It is important factors which initiate and maintain labor.

Q.7. What is lightening?

Ans. The mother experiences a sense of relief from the mechanical cardio respiratory embarrassment because presenting part sinks into the true pelvis so the fundal height is diminishes and minimizes the pressure on the diaphragm.

Q.8. What are the features of true labor pain?

Ans.
- Painful uterine contraction at regular intervals
- Contration with increasing intensity and duration
- Show
- Progressive effacement and dilation of cervix
- Formation of bag of waters.

Q.9. What are the features of false labor pain?

Ans. It appear one or two weeks prior to true labor, the features of false labor pain are:
- Dull in nature, usually confined to lower abdomen
- Continuous and unrelated with hardening of uterus
- Without any affect on dilatation of cervix
- Usually relived by enema

Reason of false pain: It occur because of taking up of cervix or may be due to stretching of cervix and lower uterine segment with consequent irritation of the neighboring ganglia.

Q.10. What is Show?

Ans. The expulsion of cervical mucus plug, mixed with blood is called show

Reason: It is slight oozing of blood from rupture of capillary vessels of the cervix and from the raw deciduas surface caused by separation of the membranes due to stretching of the lower uterine segment.

Q.11. What is the difference between contraction and retraction during labor?

Ans. **Contraction:** It is temporary reduction in length of fibers which attain their full length during relaxation

Retraction: In retraction the uterine muscle fibers are permanently shortened.

Q.12. What are the main events in first stage of labor?

Ans. The main events in first stage of labor are:

a. Dilatation and effacement of cervix
- Uterine contraction and retraction
- Bag of membranes
- Fetal axis pressure
- Vis-a-tergo

b. Full formation of lower uterine segment.

Q.13. Write the actual factor which is responsible for dilatation of cervix?

Ans.
- **Uterine contraction and retraction:** It occur in upper segment
- **Polarity of uterus:** While the upper segment contract, retracts and pushes the fetus, the lower segment and cervix dilate in response to the forces of contraction of upper segment known as polarity of uterus
- **Bag of membranes:** The membranes (amnion and chorion) are attached loosely to deciduas lining except over the internal OS. So the amniotic cavity is divided into two compartments
- **Hindwaters and forewaters:** The part above the girdle of contract contains the fetus with bulk of liquor called hindwaters and the one below it containing small amount of liquor called forewaters
- **Uterine contractions:** Generate hydrostatic pressure in the forewaters that dilate the cervical canal like a wedge
- **Fetal axis pressure:** In labor with longitudinal lie there is a tendency of straightening out of the fetal vertebral column due to contraction of circular muscle of the body of uterus hence it allows mechanical stretching of the lower segment and opening up of the cervical canal
- **Vis-a-tergo:** The dilatation and retraction of the cervix is achieved by downward thrust of presenting part of the fetus and upward pull of the cervix over the lower segment.

Q.14. What do you mean by effacement?

Ans. The muscular fibers of the cervix are pulled upward and merges with the fibers of the lower uterine segment is known as effacement.

Q.15. Define the mechanism of normal labor?

Ans. The series of movement that occur in the head in the process of adaptation, during its journey through the pelvis is called mechanism of normal labor.

Q.16. What is bearing down efforts?

Ans. It is addition voluntary expulsive efforts made by the mother to expel out the fetus that appear during the second stage of labor known as bearing down efforts and also known as expulsive phase.

Or

The expulsive force of uterine contractions is added by voluntary contraction of the abdominal muscles called "bearing down efforts"

Q.17. What is partograph?

Ans. Freidman (1954) first derived. It is graphical record of cervical dilatation and descent of head against duration of labor in hours. Also give information about fetal and maternal condition which are recorded on single sheet of paper.

Q.18. What is crowning?

Ans. The biparietal diameter stretches the vulval outlet without recession of head even after the contraction is over is called crowning of the head.

Q.19. Cervical dilatation in active phase is up to __________ cm. (10)

Q.20. Total blood loss in normal labor is __________ (380 ml)

Q.21. Cervical dilatation in latent phase is up to __________ (3 cm)

Q.22. Write the rate of dilatation in active phase per hour.

Ans. Dilatation of the cervix at the rate of 1 cm per hour in primigravidae and 1.5 cm in multigravidae beyond 3 cm dilatation is considered satisfactory.

Q.23. How you will manage first stage of labor?

Ans. Management of first stage of labor consists of:

- Non-interference with watchful expectancy
- Give encouragement, emotional support and adequate pain relief during entire course of labor
- To monitor carefully the progress of labor both maternal condition and fetal behavior
- Partograph is maintained
- The woman in labor is admitted in the hospital
- If this is the first time she is being seen, her past and present obstetric history is asked and expected date of delivery is calculated
- The vulva and perineum are clean with soap and antiseptic lotion
- Temperature, pulse rate, respiratory rate, blood pressure and fetal heart rate are recorded on admission and then every half hour
- Vaginal examination is done to see cervical dilatation and effacement, station, condition of membranes and adequacy of pelvis
- Simple soap water enema is administered if rectum is loaded with fecal matter
- Equipment necessary for delivery is arranged properly, e.g. delivery tray, instruments, gloves, sterile towels, etc.
- The patient is asked to pass urine frequently and if retention of urine, bladder should be catheterized
- A sterile pad is applied to vulva.

Q.24. Describe the second stage of labor and its management

Ans. Second stage extends from full cervical dilatation until after delivery of the baby. The membranes rupture towards the end of the first stage or beginning of the second stage of labor, so that the amniotic fluid comes out, the gravid mother bears down with uterine contractions reflex and pushes the baby out. The occiput anchors under the pubic symphysis and the fetal head delivers by extension. Then it rotates back to its original oblique position called restitution. The shoulders rotate internally and come to lie in anteroposterior diameter of the outlet that results in lateral rotation of the head called external rotation. The anterior shoulder delivers first, followed by the posterior shoulder then trunk delivers by lateral flexion.

Management

- Equipment necessary for delivery is kept near the gravida.
- Temperature, pulse rate, respiratory rate, blood pressure and fetal heart rate are recorded every 15 minutes
- If the membranes have not ruptured yet, are ruptured artificially
- Cap and mask are worn after scrubbing as for an operation, sterile gown and gloves are worn
- The gravida is put in a dorsal position and legs are drawn up
- External genitals are cleaned with Betadine. The direction of application of the swabs is from backwards. A swab is thrown away once it touches anus
- If necessary, an episiotomy is made under local anesthesia with 1% lignocaine
- The fetal head is delivered with modified Ritgens maneuvre between two uterine contractions
- If there are loops of umbilical cord around the fetal neck, they are slipped off the head either over the occiput or over the sinciput, if that fails, it is cut between two clamps
- Fetal mouth, pharynx and nose are cleaned by suction using a mucous catheter or low grade suction
- The anterior and posterior shoulders are delivered by gently pulling on the fetal head initially backward and then forward
- Apgar scoring
- Time of delivery is recorded accurately
- Injection Ergometrine is injected intravenously in a dose of 0.25 mg with the delivery of the anterior shoulder
- The umbilical cord should be clamped by two kochers forceps near on is placed 5 cm away from the umbilicus and is cut in between.

Q.25. Describe the third stage of labor and its management.

Ans. It extends from the delivery of the baby until after delivery of the placenta and membranes. It lasts for 15 minutes. The pain of uterine contraction stops in this stage.

Signs of placental separation are as follows:

- Uterine fundal height increases.
- Uterus becomes globular.
- Uterine motility from side to side increases.
- There is a gush of blood vaginally.
- There is an apparent lengthening of the umbilical cord.
- The placenta can be felt in the vagina.

Management

- The baby is held with its head down
- Its mouth, pharynx and nose are cleaned by suction
- If the baby does not cry, it is made to cry by flicking against its soles

- The placenta is removed by Brandt Andrews method, in which the uterine corpus is pushed upward and backward by suprapubic pressure, while traction is made on umbilical cord in downward direction
- Uterus is massaged abdominally until it contracts well, which arrests blood loss
- Episiotomy is sutured with no. 1-0 catgut
- The placenta and membranes are examined to see if they have been expelled completely.

Q.26. Describe the fourth stage of labor and its management.

Ans. It lasts for one hour after the third stage. The uterus remains contracted in this stage. Maternal pulse rate is slow. The mother is exhausted. There is some vaginal bleeding.

Management

- Maternal temperature, pulse rate, respiratory rate and blood pressure are recorded every 15 minutes
- The uterus is massaged abdominally periodically to keep it contracted
- Episiotomy or perineal tear, if any, is sutured with no. 1-0 chromic catgut
- Mother's private parts are cleaned
- A T-bandage is applied over a sterile pad to the vulva
- Vaginal bleeding should be watched
- Breastfeeding is started.

CHAPTER

11

Normal Puerperium

Q.1. Define puerperium?

Ans. It is the period following childbirth during which the body tissues, specially the pelvic organs revert back approximately to the pre-pregnant state both anatomically and physiologically.

Q.2. Explain the term involution.

Ans. It is the process whereby the genital organ revert back approximately to the state as were before pregnancy.

Q.3. Duration of puerperium is approximately __________ weeks after delivery. (6 weeks)

Q.4. Normal length, breadth and thickness of uterus is __________, __________ and __________ cm. (7.5 cm, 5 cm, 2.5 cm)

Q.5. Normal weight of uterus is __________ gm. (50–80)

Q.6. At term the length of uterus is __________ cm. (35)

Q.7. At puerperium the length, breadth and thickness of uterus is __________, __________ and __________ cm. (20 cm, 12 cm, 7.5)

Q.8. At term the weight of uterus is __________ gm. (1000)

Q.9. Write the endometrial changes during puerperium.

Ans. Endometrial changes occur during puerperium are:

Regeneration occurs from the epithelium completed by 10th day and the entire endometrium is restored by 16th day. Except at placental site because it takes about 6 weeks.

Q.10. What is lochia?

Ans. It is vaginal discharge for the first fortnight during puerperium. The discharge originates from the uterine body, cervix and vagina.

Q.11. What are the types of the lochia?

Ans.
- Lochia rubra (red) 1-4 days discharge
- Lochia serosa (yellowish or pink) 5–9 days discharge
- Lochia alba (pale white) 10–15 days discharge.

Q.12. The average amount of discharge for first 6 days is ______ ml. (250)

Q.13. Name the drug to improve milk production.

Ans. Metaclopramide (10 mg thrice daily) increases milk volume by increasing prolectin. Sulpuride (dopamine antagonist) has also been found effective. Intranasal oxytocin contracts myoepithelial cells and causes milk let down.

Q.14. Name the drug to suppress the lactation.

Ans. Bromocriptine that is dopamine agonist that inhibit prolectin (tab 2.5 mg) 1 tab daily for 10–14 days. Mechanical method may be used in cases where the lactation is to be suppressed after the establishment of milk secretion.

Q.15. What are the mechanical methods may be used to suppress the lactation?

Ans. The Mechanical method may be used to suppress the lactation are:

- The patient should stop breastfeeding
- She should not express out the milk from the breast
- A tight compression bandage is applied for about 2–3 days
- Analgesic tablet containing aspirin and ice packs are given to relieve pain and breast engorgement.

Q.16. What are the objectives and advantages of postnatal exercise?

Ans. The objectives and advantages of postnatal exercise are:

- To improve the muscle tone which are stretched during pregnancy and labor specially the abdominal and perineal muscles
- To educate about correct posture.

Advantages

- To minimize the risk of puerperal venous thrombosis by promoting arterial circulation and preventing venous stasis
- To prevent backache
- To prevent genital prolapsed and stress incontinence of urine.

Q.17. Which immunization should be advised if Rh negative mother bearing Rh positive baby?

Ans. Mother should immunized with anti D-gamma globulin within 24 hours after delivery.

Q.18. When steroidal contraception can be started?

Ans. It is for non-lactating women and should be started 3 weeks after delivery.

Q.19. Define postnatal care.

Ans. It includes systematic examination of the mother and the baby and appropriate advice given to the mother during postpartum period.

CHAPTER 12

Vomiting in Pregnancy

Q.1. What is morning sickness or emesis gravidarum?

Ans. Nausea and occasional sickness on rising in the morning. The vomitus is small and clear or bile stained it does not produce any impairment of health of the women is known as morning sickness.

Q.2. What is the management of morning sickness or emesis gravidarum during pregnancy?

Ans. Morning sickness manage by taking dry toast or biscuit and avoidance of fatty and spicy foods. If it fails advise antiemetic drug like trifluoperazine (Espazine) 1 mg twice daily and Phenobarbitone 30–60 mg.

Q.3. Define hyperememsis gravidarum.

Ans. It is a severe type of vomiting of pregnancy which has got deleterious effect on the health of the pregnant woman.

Q.4. Write the causes of hyperemesis gravidarum.

Ans.
- Hormonal
  - Excess of hCG
  - Progesterone excess leading to relaxation of the cardiac sphincter
- Psychogenic
- **Dietetic deficiency:** Due to low carbohydrate reserve, as it happens after a night without food
- Allergic or Immunological basis
- Decreased gastric motility is found to cause nausea
- Hydatidiform mole.

Q.5. What are the sign and symptoms of hyperemesis gravidarum?

Ans. The sign and symptoms of hyperemesis gravidarum are as follows:
- Vomiting is increased in frequency
- Urine quantity is diminished even to stage of oliguria
- Epigastric pain
- Signs of dehydration and keto-acidosis.

Q.6. How you will manage a case of hyperemesis gravidarum?

Ans. Hospitalization to the patient
- Oral feeding is withheld for at least 24 hours

- After cessation of vomiting intravenous drip should be started
- Nutrition may be given through nasogastic tube
- Antiemetic drugs-promethazine (phenargan) 25 mg or stemetil 5 mg or triflu-promazine (siquil) 10 mg may be given twice or thrice daily
- Espazine (trifluoperazine) 1 mg twice daily IM
- Metoclopramide stimulates gastric and intestinal motility without stimulating the secretions
- Nutritional support-with vitamin B_1, vitamin B_{12}, B_6 and vitamin C are given
- Diet – before the intravenous fluid is omitted, the foods are given orally. At first, dry carbohydrate foods like biscuits, bread and toast are given. Small but frequent feeds are recommended.

CHAPTER

13

Ectopic Pregnancy

Q.1. Define ectopic pregnancy.

Ans. An ectopic pregnancy is one in which the fertilized ovum is implanted and develops outside the normal uterine cavity.

Q.2. Which is the normal implantation site for fertilized ovum?

Ans. Normally fertilized ovum implanted in the endometrium of the anterior or posterior wall of the body near the fundus.

Q.3. When implantations occur?

Ans. Implantation occurs on the 6th day which corresponds to the 20th day of regular menstrual cycle.

Q.4. What are different stages of implantation of fertilized ovum?

Ans. There are mainly 4 stages of implantation:

- Apposition
- Adhesion
- Penetration
- Invasion.

Q.5. What is the abnormal site of implantation of fertilized ovum?

Ans. The abnormal site of implantation of fertilized ovum are:

Extrauterine

- Tubal-ampulla (55%)
  - Isthmus (25%)
  - Infundibulum (18%)
  - Interstitial (20%)
- Ovarian (.5%)
- Abdominal (1%)

Uterine

- Cervical
- Angular
- Cornual

Q.6. What is the risk factor of ectopic pregnancy?

Ans. History of PID

- History of tubal ligation
- Contraception failure
- Previous ectopic pregnancy
- Tubal reconstructive surgery
- History of infertility
- ART particularly if the tubes are patent but damaged
- IUD use
- Previous induced abortion.

Q.7. What are the symptoms of ectopic pregnancy?

Ans.

- **Short period of amenorrhea** of 6-8 weeks usually exceeds 10–12 weeks
- **Abdominal pain:** It is acute, agonizing or colicky in nature
- **Vaginal bleeding:** It is slight, dark colored and usually continuous bleeding
- Feeling of nausea, vomiting, fainting attacks even to the extent of syncope may be present
- **Other symptoms:** Features of bladder irritation- dysuria, frequency of urine, rise of temperature may be due to infection.

CHAPTER 14

Hemorrhage in Early Pregnancy

Q.1. What are the causes of bleeding in early pregnancy?

Ans. The causes of bleeding are broadly divided into two groups:

- Related to the pregnant state: It relates to abortion (95%), ectopic pregnancy, hydatidiform mole and implantation bleeding
- Those associated with the pregnant state: Cervical lesions as vascular erosion, polyp, ruptured varicose veins and malignancy are important causes.

Q.2. Define the abortion.

Ans. Abortion: An abortion is partial or complete separation of the products of conception from the deciduas with or without partial or complete expulsion from the genital tract before the age of viability.

Q.3. What are the causes of abortion?

Ans
- **Maternal disease:** Syphilis, high fever, toxoplasmosis, rubella, diabetes mellitus, high blood pressure, corpus luteum insufficiency, operations near the uterus
- **Diseases of the uterus:** Cervical incompetence, leiomyoma, uterine septum, bicornuate uterus
- **Foetal disease:** Germ cell defects, congenital malformations, e.g. neural tube defects.

Q.4. What are the types of abortion?

Ans.
- **Spontaneous abortion or miscarriage:** It is expulsion of embryo weighing 500 gm or less when it is not capable of independent survival
- **Threatened abortion:** It is clinical entity where the process of abortion has started but has not progressed to a state from which recovery is impossible
- **Inevitable abortion:** It is the clinical type of abortion where the changes have progressed to a state from where continuation of pregnancy is impossible
- **Complete abortion:** When the products of conception are expelled completely in mass, it is called complete abortion
- **Incomplete abortion:** When the entire products of conception are not expelled, instead a part of it is left inside the uterine cavity is called incomplete abortion
- **Missed abortion (silent miscarriage):** When the fetus is dead and retained inside the uterus for a variable period is called missed abortion

- **Recurrent miscarriage or habitual abortion:** It is defined as a sequence of three or more consecutive spontaneous abortion before 20th weeks.

Q.5. Define septic abortion, signs, symptoms, investigations and it is treatment:

Ans. Definition: When the products of conception and genital tract are infected, it is called a septic abortion.

Or

Any abortion associated with clinical evidences of infection of the uterus and its contents are called septic abortion.

Symptoms

- Amenorrhea
- Bleeding per vaginum
- Fever with chills
- Purulent discharge per vaginum
- Pain in lower abdomen.

Sign

- Fever
- Lower abdominal tenderness
- Forniceal tenderness
- Vaginal warmth
- Tender tubo-ovarian masses on one or both the sides.

Investigations

- Hemogram
- Smear, culture, antibiotic sensitivity of cervical discharge
- Urinalysis.

Treatment

- Complete bedrest in head high position
- Broad spectrum antibiotics: A combination of crystalline penicillin, gentamycin and metronidazole is used initially
- If it fails to control infection in 48 hours, higher antibiotics are used based on antibiotic sensitivity reports, e.g. cephalosporins, ciprofloxacin, etc.
- The uterus is curetted 6 hours after initiation of antibiotics therapy, if there are products of conception inside
- Sterile pad is applied to the vulva
- Sometimes the uterus has to be removed surgically.

Q.6. Define hydatidiform mole or vesicular mole.

Ans. It is an abnormal condition of the placenta where there are partly degenerative and partly proliferative changes in the young chorionic villi.

Q.7. Describe the symptoms, signs and management of a vesicular mole. What is it's complication?

Ans. Vesicular mole is a gestational trophoblastic neoplasm that develops from the placenta.

Symptoms

- Amenorrhea,
- Excessive nausea and vomiting,
- Bleeding per vaginum which could be severe,
- Fetal movements are not felt,
- Edema on feet before 20th weeks of pregnancy.

Signs

- Pregnancy induced hypertension before 20 completed weeks of pregnancy
- Uterine size is more than expected for the period of amenorrhea
- Uterus feels tense and cystic
- External ballottement is absent
- Internal ballottement is absent
- Fetal parts cannot be felt
- Fetal heart sounds cannot be heard
- Anemia.

Investigations

- Pregnancy test on urine: If it is positive in a dilution of 1:200 or more, the diagnosis is confirmed
- Plasma beta hCG levels are more than 1000 lu/ml thereafter
- Ultrasonography shows a snow storm appearance in the uterus and no fetal shadow
- Hysterography, angiography are not done though useful for diagnosis because they are dangerous
- Hemoglobin
- Blood group.

Treatment

- If the bleeding is excessive, or if the patient is in shock, intravenous infusion of ringer lactate and blood transfusion are given
- Vulva is shaved and a sterile pad is applied to it
- Temperature, pulse rate, respiratory rate, blood pressure and fundal height of the woman are recorded every half hour, and vaginal bleeding is watched
- The vesicular mole is removed by rapid dilatation and suction evacuation. Check curettage is done and the material is sent for histopathological examination
- Methyl ergometrine, oxytocin or prostaglandin is used to achieve uterine contraction and stop bleeding

- If beta-hCG is present is her urine 60 days after evacuation, or if its levels are rising. antimalignancy chemotherapy is given with methotrexate or actinomycin-D.

Postevacuation management

- The patient should see the doctor if there is abnormal bleeding per vaginum
- Contraception in the form of a condom or combination contraceptive pills is used for one year
- Urine and blood are checked every week until they show absence of beta-BCG.
- Methotrexate or actinomycin-D is used as required.

Complications

- Hemorrhage
- Shock
- Uterine sepsis
- Pregnancy induced hypertension
- Choriocarcinoma
- Thyrotoxicosis.

CHAPTER 15

Multiple Pregnancies

Q.1. Define multiple pregnancies.

Ans. When more than one fetus simultaneously develops in the uterus it is called multiple pregnancies.

Q.2. What are different varieties of twins?

Ans. It is two types:

- **Dizygotic twins:** Result from fertilization of two ova most likely ruptured from two distinct grafian follicles usually same or one from each ovary, by two sperms during a single ovarian cycle
- **Monozygotic twins (identical or uniovular):** The twinning may occur at different periods after fertilization. There is varying degree of free anastomosis between the two fetal vessels.

Q.3. What is the common complication of twin pregnancy?

Ans. Maternal complication during pregnancy:

- Nausea and vomiting
- Anaemia: Due to increase iron and folate requirement
- Pre-eclampsia: May be due to overdistension of uterus
- Hydramnious
- Antepartum hemorrhage
- Malpresentation
- Preterm labor
- Mechanical distress.

During labor

- Early rupture of membranes and cord prolapsed
- Prolonged labor
- Bleeding
- Postpartum hemorrhage.

During puerperium

- Subinvolution-due to bigger size of uterus

- Infection-due to increased operative interferance
- Lactation failure.

Fetal

- Growth problem
- Intrauterine death of one fetus in monozygotic
- Fetal anomalies
- Asphyxia and stillbirth
- Loscked twins.

Q.4. Why placenta previa occur as complication in twin pregnancy?
Ans. It is because of bigger size of placenta encroaching on to the lower segment.

Q.5. Why hydramnios is more in monozygotic twins?
Ans. It is because of increased urinary output which may accompany the hypervolemia in the larger twin.

Q.6. Iron requirement in twin pregnancy is _________ mg/day. (60–100)

Q.7. Define polyhydramnios?
Ans. A state where liquor amnii exceeds 2000 ml.
In USG- when amniotic fluid index (AFI) is more than 25 cm and single pool is > 8 cm.

Q.8. What are the causes of polyhydramnios?
Ans. Fetal anomalies-

- Anencephaly
- Open spina bifida
- Esophageal or duodenal atresia
- Facial clefts and neck masses
- Hydrops fetalis
  - Placental cause due to chorioangioma of placenta: Tumour in single villus consisting of hyperplasia of blood vessels and connective tissue results in increasing transudation
  - Multiple pregnancy
  - Maternal cause diabetes: It is due to raised maternal blood sugar→raised fetal blood sugar→fetal divresis →hydramnios.

Q.9. How fetal anomalies like anencephaly are responsible for polyhydramnios?
Ans. It is due to:

- Transudation from the exposed meninges.
- Absence of fetal swallowing reflex.

Possible suppression of fetal antidiuretic hormone leading to excessive urination.

Q.10. Define oligohydramnios.
Ans. The condition where the liquor amnii is deficient in amount to the extent of less than 200 ml at term.

Q.11. Write the causes of oligohydramnios.

Ans. Still the cause of oligohydramnios is not known but it associated with following factors:

- Fetal chromosomal anomalies
- Intrauterine infection
- Drugs-prostaglandine inhibitors
- IUGR associated with placental insufficiency
- Postmaturity.

Q.12. Write about abnormalities of cord.

Ans.
- Battlledore placenta: The cord is attached to the margin of the placenta.
- Velamentous placenta: The cord is attached to the membranes.

Q.13. Write the treatment of abnormal cord.

Ans. In case of fetal bleeding, urgent delivery is essential either vaginally or caesarean section.

Q.14. Single umbilical artery is present in ______ and in babies born of __________ or in _______. (twin, diabetic mother, polyhyramnios)

CHAPTER

16

Hypertensive Disorders in Pregnancy

Q.1. Classify the hypertensive disorders in pregnancy.

Ans.

A. Gestational hypertension:
   - Without proteinuria or pathological edema.

B. Pre-eclampsia
   - Hypertension and proteinuria with or without pathological edema.

C. Eclampsia: pre–eclampsia with convulsion or coma.

D. Chronic hypertension
   - Essential hypertension
   - Chronic renal disease
   - Coarctation of aorta
   - Pheochromocytoma
   - Thyrotoxicosis
   - Connective tissue disease—systemic lupus erythematous.

Q.2. Define Pre-eclampsia.

Ans. Pre-eclampsia is a multi system disorder of unknown etiology characterized by development of hypertension to the extent of 140/90 mm of Hg or more with proteinuria after the 20th weeks in a previously normotensive and non-proteinuric patient.

Q.3. In which condition pre-eclamptic features may be appear before 20th weeks of gestation?

Ans. In case of hydatidiform mole and acute polyhydromnios, pre-eclamptic features may be appear before 20th weeks.

Q.4. What are the diagnostic criteria of Pre-eclampsia?

Ans.

- **Hypertension:** An absolute rise of blood pressure at least 140/90 mm of Hg of raise in systolic pressure of at least 30 mm of Hg or rise in diastolic pressure of at least 15 mm of Hg.
- **Edema:** Pitting edema over the ankles after 12 hrs. Bed rest or rapid gain in weight of more than 1lb a week or more than 5 lb a month in the later month of pregnancy.
- **Proteinuria:** Presence of total protein in 24 hours urine of more than 0·3 gm on at least two random clean catch urine samples.

Q.5. What are the risk factors of Pre-eclampsia?

Ans. **a.** Primigravida–young and elderly.

b. Family history-hypertension, pre-eclampsia, eclampsia.

c. Placental abnormalities-poor placentation, hyperplacentosis, molar pregnancy, genetic disorder.

d. Placental ischemia.

e. Immunologic phenomenon.

f. New paternity.

g. Pre-existing vascular and renal disease.

Q.6. What are the alarming symptoms of Pre-eclampsia?

Ans. Headache-either located over the occipital or frontal region

- Disturbed sleep
- Diminished urinary output—Urinary output less than 400 ml in 24 hours
- Epigastric pain—Acute pain in epigastric region associated with vomiting
- Eye symptoms—There may be blurring or dimness of vision or at times complete blindness. Vision is usually regained within 4–6 weeks following delivery.

Q.7. What are the signs of Pre-eclampsia?

Ans. Rapid weight gain—Weight gains more than 5 lb a month or more than 1 lb a week in later month of pregnancy.

- Rise of blood pressure.
- Edema.
- Pulmonary edema-due to leaky capillaries and low oncotic pressure.

Q.8. A serum uric acid level of more than ________ mg/dl indicates the presence of pre-eclampsia. (4·5)

Q.9. What is the complication of eclampsia?

Ans. Maternal complication is:

- Eclampsia
- Shock
- Sepsis.

Fetal complication are:

- Intrauterine death.
- Intrauterine growth restriction.
- Asphyxia
- Prematurity.

Q.10. How to prevent pre-eclampsia in high-risk group of patient?

Ans. Regular antenatal checkup—Detection for weight gain, rise of diastolic pressure, rise in uric acid level.

- Antithrombotic agents—low dose aspirine 60 mg daily is reduces platelet thromboxane production.
- Calcium supplementation (2 gm/day) reduces the risk of pre-eclampsia.
- Antioxidants, vit E and C, taking from 16–22 weeks onwards reduce the risk of pre-eclampsia.

- Nutritional supplementation—With magnesium, zinc, fish oil, high protein and low salt diet has been tried but are of limited benefit.

Q.11. Write the management of the pre-eclampsia.

Ans.
- **Rest:** Admission in hospital. Advise the patient to take rest and while in bed patient should be in left lateral position because it lesser the effects of venacaval compression
- **Diet:** It should contain adequate amount of protein about 100 gm usual salt intake is not restricted. Fluids need not be restricted
- **Sedative:** To cut down emotion phenobarbitone 60 mg or diazepam 5 mg at bedtime
- **Diuretics:** Frusemide (lasix) 40 mg given orally after breakfast for 5 days in a week
- Antihypertensives drugs
  - Labetalol 200 mg in 200 ml of normal saline
  - Hydralazine 5 mg bolus in infusion 25 mg in 200 ml normal saline
  - Nitroglycerin 5 micro gm/mins.

Q.12. Define eclampsia.

Ans. When pre-eclampsia complicated with convulsion is called Eclampsia.

Q.13. How rest helps in reducing blood pressure in pre-eclampsia?

Ans. Rest increases the renal blood flow that leads to diuresis.

It also increases the uterine blood flow that improves the placental perfusion and it reduces the blood pressure.

Q.14. What are the causes of convulsion in eclampsia?

Ans. The causes of cerebral irritation leads to convulsion is not clear, causes of irritation may be provoked by:

a. Anoxia—Due to spasm of cerebral vessels following hypertension that increased cerebral vascular resistance that causes fall in cerebral oxygen consumption lead to anoxia.

b. Cerebral edema— It contribute to irritation.

c. Cerebral dysrhythmia— Increases following anoxia.

Q.15. What are the different stages of eclampsia?

Ans. It consists of four stages:
- **Premonitory stage:** There is twitching of the muscles of the face, tongue and limbs, eye balls roll or turned to one side and become fixed. This stage lasts for 30 seconds
- **Tonic stage:** Tonic spasm present on whole body. Limbs are flexed and hands clenched. Respiration ceases and tongue protrudes between teeth. Cyanosis appears Eye balls become fixed. It last for about 30 seconds
- **Clonic stage:** All voluntary muscles undergo alternate contraction and relaxation. The twitching start in the face then involves one side of the extremities and ultimately whole body is involved in the convulsion. Biting of the tongue occurs. This stage lasts for 1–4 minutes

- Stage of coma: Following the fit the patient passes on the stage of coma. On occasion the patient appears to be in a confused state following the fit and fails to remember the happenings.

Q.16. What is the general management of patient with eclampsia?

Ans. Patient should be placed in a railed cot in an isolated room.

- Half hourly pulse, respiration rate and blood pressure to be recorded. Immediately after a convulsion, fetal bradycardia is common probably due to maternal acidosis and hypoxia induced by the fit
- **Fluid balance:** Ringer solution is started the total fluids should not exceed the previous 24 hours urinary output plus 1000 ml. Normally it should not exceed 2 litres in 24 hours
- **Antibiotics:** To prevent infection. Injection Ampicillin 500 mg IM or IV six hourly is administered.

Q.17. What management we should perform during fits?

Ans. In the premonitory stage: A mouth gag is placed in between the teeth to prevent tongue bite and it should be remove over clonic phase.

- The air passage should be clear. Patient head should be turned to one side and pillow is taken off
- Raising the footend of bed it facilitates postural drainage of upper respiratory tract
- Oxygen is given until cyanosis is disappears.

Q.18. What is Gestational Hypertension?

Ans. A sustained rise of blood pressure to 140/90 mm of Hg or more on at least two occasions or more hours apart beyond the 20th week of pregnancy or during the first 24 hours after delivery in a previously normotensive woman is called gestational hypertension.

Q.19. Define chronic hypertension disease.

Ans. Chronic hypertensive disease is defined as the presence of hypertension of any cause before 20th week of pregnancy and its presence beyond the 42 days after delivery.

Q.20. What are the specific congenital or acquired cardiac lesions?

Ans. Specific congenital or acquired cardiac lesions can be classified as low, intermediate, or high-risk during pregnancy.

Q.21. What are low risk of maternal cardiac lesions and cardiac complications during pregnancy?

Ans. Low risk cardiac complications during pregnancy are:

- Atrial septal defect
- Ventricular septal defect
- Patent ductus arteriosus
- Asymptomatic AS with low mean gradient (< 50 mm Hg) and normal LV function (EF > 50%)
- AR with normal LV function and NYHA Class I or II
- MVP (Isolated or with mild or moderate MR and normal LV function)

- MR with normal LV function and NYHA Class I or II Mild or moderate MS (MVA > 1.5 cm^2, mean gradient < 5 mm Hg) without severe pulmonary hypertension.

Q.22. What are intermediate risk of maternal cardiac lesions and cardiac complications during pregnancy?

Ans. Maternal cardiac lesions and intermediate risk of cardiac complications during pregnancy are:

- Large left to right shunt
- Coarctation of the aorta
- Marfan syndrome with a normal aortic root
- Moderate or severe MS
- Mild or moderate AS and Severe PS.

Q.23. What are high risk of maternal cardiac lesions and cardiac complications during pregnancy?

Ans. High Risk are:

- Eisenmenger's syndrome
- Severe pulmonary hypertension
- Complex cyanotic heart disease (TOF, Ebstein's anomaly, TA, TGA, tricuspid atresia)
- Marfan syndrome with aortic root or valve involvement
- Severe AS with or without symptoms
- Aortic or mitral valve disease or both (stenosis or regurgitation) with moderate or severe LV dysfunction (EF < 40%)
- NYHA Class III or IV symptoms associated with any valvular disease or with cardiomyopathy of any cause
- History of prior peripartum cardiomyopathy.

Q.24 What is the drug therapy of hypertension in Pregnancy?

Ans. Drug Therapy of Hypertension in Pregnancy

First line

- Alpha methyldopa (PO)
- Labetolol (PO).

Second Line

- Hydralazine (PO)
- Nifedipine (PO)
- Beta blockers (PO).

Contraindicated

- Angiotensin-converting enzyme inhibitors (PO)
- Angiotensin receptor blockers (PO)
- Aldosterone antagonists (PO)

Avoid

- Thiazide diuretics

Severe Hypertensive Urgency or Emergency First Line

- Labetolol (IV)
- Hydralazine (IV)

- Beta blockers (IV)
- Nifedipine (PO).

Q.25. What are the possible risk and complications of cesarean section?

Ans. A cesarean section is a relatively common and comparatively safe surgical procedure. However, as with all surgical procedures, there are risks for both mother and baby. Some of these risks and possible complications include:

- Infection of the mother's wounds
- Damage to the mother's bladder and other internal organs
- Damage to the mother's blood vessels
- Damage to the baby inflicted by surgical instruments
- Increased risk of the baby experiencing respiratory distress (breathing problems) after birth
- Increased time in hospital
- Increased abdominal (tummy) pain
- Increased risk of blood clots
- Increased risk of the placenta growing or implanting too low in the uterus or through the uterus in future pregnancies
- Increased risk of having a cesarean section with future pregnancies.

Q.26. Write the types of incisions of cesarean section.

Ans. There are two types of incisions (cuts) in the uterus:

A lower segment incision: This is a horizontal (across) cut through the abdomen (tummy) and a horizontal cut through the lower part of the uterus, sometimes known as a bikini line incision. These cuts heal better are less visible and are less likely to cause problems in future pregnancies.

A classical incision: Refers to a vertical incision on the uterus. The incision on the abdomen (tummy) may be horizontal or vertical. These days this incision is common only for extreme emergencies or in specific situations, such as if the placenta is lying very low, if baby is lying sideways or if baby is very small. The chance of problems is greater in subsequent pregnancies when this kind of incision is used.

Elective or emergency cesarean there are two types of cesarean section:

Elective: A cesarean section is called elective. If it decides is necessary before labor begins.

Emergency: A cesarean section is called emergency. If it decides is necessary after labor has begun.

CHAPTER 17

Episiotomy

Q.1. Define episiotomy.

Ans. A surgically planned incision on the perineum and the posterior vaginal wall during second stage of labor. The incision, which can be midline or at an angle from the posterior end of the vulva.

Q.2. What is the indication of episiotomy?

Ans. Indications are:

- There is a serious risk to the mother of second or third degree tearing
- In cases where a natural delivery is adversely affected, but a Caesarean section is not indicated
- Natural tearing will cause an increased risk of maternal disease being vertically transmitted
- When baby is very large
- When perineal muscles are excessively rigid
- When instrumental delivery is indicated
- When a woman has undergone FGM (female genital mutilation), indicating the need for an anterior and or mediolateral episiotomy
- Prolonged late decelerations or fetal bradycardia during active pushing
- The baby's shoulders are stuck (shoulder dystocia), or a bony association.

Q.3. What are the types of episiotomy?

Ans. **Medio–lateral:** The incision is made from midpoint of fourchette either to right or left. It is directed diagonally in straight line which runs about 2.5 cm away from the anus (midpoint between anus and ischial tuberosity).

- **Median:** The incision commences from center of the fourchette and extends on posterior side along midline for 2.5 cm
- **Lateral:** The incision starts from about 1 cm away from the center of fourchette and extends laterally. Drawback includes chance of injury to Bartholin's duct. Thus some practioners have totally condemned it
- **J shaped:** The incision begins in the center of the fourchette and is directed posteriorly along midline for about 1.5 cm and then directed downwards and outwards along 5 or 7 o'clock position to avoid the anal sphincter.

CHAPTER 18

Hematological Disorders in Pregnancy Anemia in Pregnancy

Q.1. Write the classification of anemia.

Ans. i. **Deficiency anemia**
- Iron deficiency
- Folic acid deficiency
- Vitamin B12 deficiency
- Protein deficiency.

ii. **Haemorrhagic**
- Acute-antepartum hemorrhage
- Chronic- hookworm infestation and bleeding piles, etc.

iii. **Hereditary**
- Thalassemias, sickle cell hemoglobinopathies
- Hereditary hemolytic anemias.

iv. **Bone marrow insufficiency**
- Aplasia due to radiation, drug (aspirin, indomethacin).

v. **Anemia of infection (malaria, tuberculosis).**

vi. **Chronic renal disease.**

Q.2. What are the criteria of physiological anemia during pregnancy?

Ans. The lower limit of physiological anemia during the second half of pregnancy should be fulfill the following hematological values- If:
- Hb 10 gm%
- RBC-3·2 million/mm^3
- PCV-30%
- Peripherral smear showing normal morphology of RBC with central pallor.

Q.3. The average life span of red cells is about _________ days. (120)

Q.4. What is normal erythropoiesis?

Ans. In adults erythropoiesis is confined to the bone marrow. Red blood cells are formed through stages of pronormoblasts → normoblasts→ reticulocytes → to mature non- nucleated erythrocytes. After 120 days the RBC degenerate and hemoglobin is broken down into hemosiderin and bile pigment. For proper erythropoiesis, adequate nutrients are needed.

Q.5. What are the complication of severe anemia?

Ans. • During pregnancy
- Pre-eclampsia

  - Intercurrent infection
  - Heart failure
  - Preterm labor.
- During labor
  - Uterine inertia
  - Postpartum hemorrhage is a real threat
  - Cardiac failure
  - Shock.
- Puerperium
  - Puerperal sepsis
  - Subinvolution
  - Failing lactation
  - Puerperal venous thrombosis
  - Pulmonary embolism.

Q.6. What are the features and symptoms of Iron deficiency anemia?

Ans. In majority of patient have no symptoms but the symptoms are lassitude and feeling of exhaustion or weakness, anorexia, indigestion, palpitation caused by ectopic beats, dyspnea, giddiness and swelling of the legs.

Q.7. How will you treat the patient with anemia?

Ans. Prophylactic Treatment

- Avoidance of frequent child births.
- Supplementary iron therapy- 200 mg of ferrous sulfate along with 1 mg folic acid.
- Tea should be avoided within one hour of taking iron tablet.
- Dietary prescription- Diet should be rich in iron and protein that should be easily digestible like liver, meat, egg, green vegetables, green peas, gigs, beans, whole wheat and onion stalks, jaggery, etc.
- Iron utensils should preferably be used for cooking.
- Adequate treatment to eradicate hookworm infestation, dysentery, malaria, bleeding piles and UTI.

Curative treatment- Diet rich in protein, iron and vitamins.

- To improve appetite and facilitate digestion- preparation containing acid pepsin may be given.
- To eradicate even a minimal septic focus.
- Iron therapy- oral therapy and parenteral iron therapy.

Q.8. What are the complication of severe anemia?

Complication of severe anemia are:

Ans. During pregnancy

a. Pre-eclampsia
b. Intercurrent infection
c. Heart failure
d. Preterm labor.

During labor

a. Uterine inertia
b. Postpartum hemorrhage is a real threat
c. Cardiac failure
d. Shock.

Puerperium

a. Puerperal sepsis
b. Subinvolution
c. Failing lactation
d. Puerperal venous thrombosis
e. Pulmonary embolism.

Q.9 Write about the oral iron therapy and parenteral iron therapy.

Ans. Oral iron therapy

Preparation are ferrous gluconate, ferrous fumarate or ferrous sulfate that contain 200 mg ferrous sulfate which contain 60 mg of elemental iron and trace of coper and maganacese.

The initial dose 1 tab thrice daily with after meals. It should be stepped up gradually in three to four days, there- after maintenance dose one tab daily is to be continued for at least 100 days following delivery to replenish the iron stores.

Parenteral iron therapy

Estimation of total requirement
= 0·3 weight (100-Hb %)
W = weight in pounds
= 0·3 100 (100-50)
= 3/10 100 50 = 1500 mg and add 50% additional that is 750 mg for partial replenishment of body store iron
1500 + 750 = 2250 mg.

Q.10. All women of reproductive age should be given ______ of folic acid daily. (400 µg)

Q.11. Define the megaloblastic Anemia.

Ans. In megaloblastic anaemia there is dearrengement in red cell maturation with the production in the bone marrow of abnormal precursors known as megaloblasts due to impaired DNA synthesis or due to deficiency of vitamin B12 or folate both.

Q.12. The daily requirement of vit B12 in non-pregnant condition is ___µg. (2)

Q.13. The daily requirement of vit B12 in pregnancy is ________ µg. (3)

Q.14. Define aplastic anemia.

Ans. It is rarely seen in pregnancy there is marked decrease in the bone marrow stem cells or it may be immunologically mediated or may be an autosomal recessive inheritance.

Q.15. Explain the NYHA (New York Heart Association) classification of heart disease?

Ans. Grade I: uncompromised— Patient with cardiac disease but no limitation of physical activity.

Grade II: slightly compromised— Patient with cardiac disease with slight limitation of physical activity.

The patients are comfortable at rest but ordinary physical activity causes discomfort.

Grade III: Markedly compromise—Patients with cardiac disease with marked limitation of activity. The patients are comfortable at rest but discomforts occur with less than ordinary activity.

Grade IV: Severely compromised— Patient with cardiac disease with discomfort even at rest.

CHAPTER

19

Antepartum Hemorrhage

Q.1. Define antepartum hemorrhage.

Ans. It is defined as bleeding from or into genital tract after the 28th weeks of pregnancy but before the birth of the baby.

Q.2. What are the causes of antepartum hemorrhage?

Ans.
- Placental bleeding—
  - Placenta previa (35%)
  - Abruptio placentae (35%)
- Unexplained (25%) - placental bleeding and local lesions
- Extra placental causes (5%) - local cervicovaginal lesions
  - Cervical polyp
  - Carcinoma cervix
  - Varicose vein
  - Local trauma.

Q.3. Define placenta previa.

Ans. When the placenta is implanted partially or completely over the lower uterine segment it is called Placenta previa.

Q.4. What are the different theories are postulated for implantation of placenta?

Ans.
- Dropping down theory—The fertilized ovum drops down and is implanted in lower segment due to poor decidual reaction in upper segment
- Persistent of chorionic activity
- Defective deciduas: Due to spreading of the chorionic villi over a wide area in the uterine wall to get nourishment. In this process, not only the placenta becomes membranous but encroaches into the lower segment. Such placenta previa may invade the underlying deciduas to cause placenta accreta or percreta
- Big surface area of the placenta as in twins may encroach into the lower segment.

Q.5. What are the predisposing factors for placenta previa?

Ans.
- Multiparity.
- Increased maternal age (>35 years).
- History of previous cesarean section or any other scar in uterus.
- Placental size and abnormality.
- Smoking causes placental hypertrophy to compensate carbon monoxide induced hypoxemia.

Q.6. What are the types of degrees of Placenta previa?

Ans. There are four types of placenta previa depending upon the degree of extension of placenta to lower segment.

- **Type I:** Major part of placenta is attached to upper segment and only the lower margin encroaches into the lower segment but not up to the os
- **Type II:** (Marginal) - The placenta reaches the margin of internal os but does not cover it
- **Type III:** (Incomplete or partial central): The placenta covers the internal os partially
- **Type IV:** (Central or total): The placenta completely covers the internal os of even after full dilatation.

Q.7. Which one is given name as Dangerous Placenta previa and why?

Ans. Type II posterior placenta previa is more dangerous because—

- The curved birth canal major thickness of the placenta (2·5 cm) overlies the sacral promontory, thereby diminishing the anteroposterior diameter of the inlet and prevents engagement of the presenting part
- Placenta is more likely to be compressed if vaginal delivery is allowed
- More chance of cord compression or cord prolapsed
- It may produce fetal anoxia or even fetal death.

Q.8. Why bleeding occur in placenta previa?

Ans. As the placental growth slows down in later months and the lower segment progressively dilates the inelastic placenta is sheared off the wall of the lower segment. This leads to opening up of utero-placental vessels and leads to an episode of bleeding.

Q.9. How bleeding is spontaneously control in placenta previa?

Ans. Bleeding is spontaneously control due to following reason:

- Thrombosis of the open sinuses
- Mechanical pressure by the presenting part
- Placental infarction.

Q.10. Which type of bleeding occurs in placenta previa?

Ans. The bleeding of placenta preavia will sudden onset, painless, apparently causeless and recurrent.

Q.11. Bright red vaginal bleeding occur in __________. (Placenta previa)

Q.12. What is the management of placenta previa?

Ans. All APH patients should be admitted for

- Expectant treatment
  - If no active bleeding
  - Pregnancy 37 weeks
  - Patient stable and FHS good
  - Internal examination in OT if Type I,II (anterior placenta previa)

ARM should be done with oxytocin if satisfactory progress without any bleeding allow for vaginal delivery. If bleeding coutinues – cesarean section should be done. In case of Type II (post), III and IV- cesarean section should be done.

Active interference-- When bleeding is continues, pregnancy > 37 weeks, patient in labor, FHS absent, gross fetal malformation than without internal examination CS should be performed.

Q.13. Define abruptio placentae.

Ans. It is one of antepartum hemorrhage where the bleeding occurs due to premature separation of normally situated placenta after the 20th week of gestation and prior to birth.

Q.14. What are the different varieties of abruption placentae?

Ans. It is three types:

a. **Revealed:** Blood comes out of the cervical canal to be visible externally. It is common.

c. **Concealed:** The blood collects behind the separated placenta between the membranes and decidua. In any of the circumstances blood is not visible outside. It is rare type.

c. **Mixed:** Some part of blood collects inside and a part of blood is expelled out this is quite common.

Prevalence is more with:

a. High birth order.
b. Advancing age of mother.
c. Poor socioeconomic condition.
d. Malnutrition, smoking.

Q.15. What are the causes of abruptio placentae?

Ans. Exact cause is obscure but following factors are responsible for abruption placenta:

a. Hypertension in pregnancy- When spasm of the vessels in utero placental bed leads to anoxic endothelial damage cause rupture of vessels in the deciduas basalis
b. Trauma
c. Sudden uterine decompression
d. Short cord- During labor by mechanical pull
e. Supine hypotension syndrome
f. Sick placenta
g. Folic acid deficiency
h. Torsion of the uterus
i. Cocain abuse, thrombophilias.

Q.16. What are factors that increase the risk for placental abruption and what may be the maternal and fetal complications?

Ans. The following factors are among those that increase the risk for placental abruption:

- Maternal hypertension
- Maternal trauma
- Association with domestic violence
- Smoking habit
- Substance abuse
- Advanced maternal age

- Premature ruptured membranes
- Uterine fibromyomas
- Amniocentesis.

Potential maternal complications include the following:

- Hemorrhagic shock
- Coagulopathy/disseminated intravascular coagulation (DIC)
- Uterine rupture
- Renal failure
- Ischemic necrosis of distal organs (e.g. hepatic, adrenal, pituitary).

Potential fetal complications include the following:

- Hypoxia
- Anemia
- Growth retardation
- CNS anomalies
- Fetal death.

CHAPTER

20

Cephalopelvic Disproportion

Q.1. Define the cephalopelvic disproportion.

Ans. Cephalopelvic disproportion is disproportion in relation between the head of baby and pelvis of mother.

Q.2. What are the risks of CPD?

Ans. To mother:

- Prolonged and painful labor
- Failure of the cervix to dilate
- Failure of fetal descends with resultant need for operative delivery
- Uterine rupture from prolonged thinning of lower uterine segment during non-progressive but active labor process.

To fetus:

- Extensive caput and moulding from the prolonged labor
- Fetal intolerance with resultant hypoxia from prolonged labor

Potential for birth injury related to difficult and traumatic delivery.

Q.3. Write the management of cephalopelvic disproportion.

Ans. Minor degrees of inlet contraction do not give rise to problems and have spontaneous vaginal delivery at term.

The moderate and severe degrees are managed by one of the following methods.

- **Premature induction of labor:** This is limited only to moderate degree of disproportion in selected multigravidae, 2–3 weeks prior to due date.
- **Elective caesarean section at term:** This is indicated in major degree of inlet contraction associated with outlet contraction or complicating factors like elderly primigravida, malpresentation, postmaturity toxemia and post caesarean delivery is known, the operation is planned and done in the last week of pregnancy. In cases where fetal maturity is not known, the operation is withheld till labor pains start maturity is not known or the membranes rupture, whatever occurs early.

  Trial of labor: This is the preferred management method for a client with minor degree of cephalopelvic disproportion at the inlet.

Q.4. What are the advantages of trial labor?

Ans. • Eliminates unnecessary caesarean section electively decided.

- A successful outcome leading to a vaginal delivery secures the client's obstetric future.

  A successful trial ensures the woman a good future obstetrics.

Q.5. What are the disadvantages of trial labor?

Ans.
- Caesarean section may have to be performed for about half of the cases because of fetal distress of abnormal uterine action
- Fetal morbidity and mortality may be higher than with elective caesarean section
- Maternal morbidity is higher

When trial fails and the client has to face a surgical procedure, she is disappointed, dehydrated, frightened and in poor shape.

Q.6. What are the contraindications of trial labor?

Ans.
- Severe disproportion, true conjugate less than 9 cm
- If in a previous pregnancy, trial of labor had failed
- Maternal diseases like diabetes, pregnancy induced hypertension, cardiac condition
- Intrauterine growth restriction
- Cases of malpresentation, e.g. breech
- Previous caesarean section.

Q.7. Define prolonged labor.

Ans. The labor is said to be prolonged when the combined duration of the first and second stage is more than the arbitrary time limit of 18 hours.

Q.8. Normal duration of latent phase is about __________ hours in a primi and __________ hours observation. (8 hrs and 4 hrs)

Q.9. What are the causes of prolonged latent phase in prolonged labor?

Ans. The causes include
- Unripe cervix
- Malposition and malpresentation
- Cephalopelvic disproportion
- Premature rupture of the membranes.

Q.10. What are the causes of prolonged labor?

Ans. Failure to dilate the cervix is due to:
- **Fault in power:** Uterine inertia or incoordination uterine contraction
- **Fault in the passage:** Contracted pelvis, cervical dystocia, pelvic tumor or even full bladder
- **Fault in the passenger:** Malposition and malpresentation, congenital anomalies of the fetus
- **Others:** Early administration of sedatives and analgesics before the active labor begins.

Q.11. What is the management of prolonged labor?

Ans. Management of prolonged labor are:
- Reassessment of the condition

- Pain relief: Pethidine or epidural analgesia
- Amniotomy: If membranes still intact
- Oxytocin: If amniotomy does not bring good uterine contractions and there is no contraindication for it.

Caesarean section is indicated in:

- Failure of the above measures
- Disproportion
- Malpresentations not amenable for vaginal delivery
- Contraindications to oxytocin
- Fetal distress.

Q.12. What are the causes of prolonged labor?

Ans. Prolonged or obstructed labor may be due to one of the 'Ps' that is 'powers', 'passenger' and 'passage'.

- **Powers:** Inadequate power, due to poor or uncoordinated uterine contractions, is a major cause of prolonged labor.
- Either the uterine contractions are not strong enough to efface and dilate the cervix in the first stage of labor.
- The muscular effort of the uterus is insufficient to push the baby down through birth canal during the second stage.
- **Passenger:** The fetus is the 'passenger' travelling down the birth canal.
- Prolonged labor may occur if the fetal head is too large to pass through the mother's pelvis or the fetal presentation is abnormal.
- **Passage:** The birth canal is the passage, so labor may be prolonged if the mother's pelvis is too small for the baby to pass through or the pelvis has an abnormal shape or if there is a tumor or other physical obstruction in the pelvis.

Causes of passenger and passage failures that lead to prolonged and possibly obstructed labors.

Passenger	Passage
Head:	***Bony pelvis:***
• Large fetal head (big for that pelvis)	• Contracted (due to malnutrition)
• Hydrocephalus (brain surrounded by fluid, which makes the skull swell)	• Deformed (due to trauma, polio)
Presentation and position:	***Soft tissue:***
• Brow, face, shoulder	• Tumor in the pelvis
• Persistent malposition	• Viral infection in the uterus or abdomen
Twin pregnancy:	
• Locked twins (locked at the neck)	• Scars (from female circumcision)
• Conjoined twins (fused together with some shared organs)	

CHAPTER 21

Gestational Diabetes

Q.1. What is gestational diabetes?

Ans. This is a type of diabetes that some women get during pregnancy.

- Diabetes is high levels of sugar in blood. When digestive system breaks most of food down into a type of sugar called glucose. The glucose enters bloodstream and then, with the help of insulin (a hormone made by pancreas), cells use the glucose as fuel. However, body does not produce enough insulin or cells have a problem responding to the insulin – too much glucose remains in blood instead of moving into the cells and getting converted to energy
- When hormonal changes can make cells less responsive to insulin. For most moms-to-be, this is not a problem: When the body needs additional insulin, the pancreas dutifully secretes more of it. But if pancreas cannot keep up with the increased insulin demand during pregnancy, blood glucose levels rise too high, resulting in gestational diabetes
- Most women with gestational diabetes do not remain diabetic after the baby is born. Once gestational diabetes occurred though, women at higher risk for getting it again during a future pregnancy and for developing diabetes later in life.

Q.2. Define gestational diabetes.

Ans. Gestational diabetes is a condition characterized by high blood sugar (glucose) levels that is first recognized during pregnancy. The condition occurs in approximately 4% of all pregnancies.

Q.3. What is pathophysiology of Gestational Diabetes in pregnancy?

Ans. Almost all women have some degree of impaired glucose intolerance as a result of hormonal changes that occur during pregnancy. That means the blood sugar may be higher than normal, but not high enough to have diabetes. During the later part of pregnancy (the third trimester), these hormonal changes place pregnant woman at risk for gestational diabetes.

During pregnancy, increased levels of certain hormones made in the placenta (the organ that connects the baby by the umbilical cord to the uterus) help shift nutrients from the mother to the developing fetus. Other hormones are produced by the placenta to help prevent the mother from developing low blood sugar. They work by stopping the actions of insulin.

Over the course of the pregnancy, these hormones lead to progressive impaired glucose intolerance (higher blood sugar levels). To try to decrease blood sugar levels, the body makes more insulin to get glucose into cells to be used for energy.

Usually the mother's pancreas is able to produce more insulin (about three times the normal amount) to overcome the effect of the pregnancy hormones on blood sugar levels. If, however, the pancreas cannot produce enough insulin to overcome the effect of the increased hormones during pregnancy, blood sugar levels will rise, resulting in gestational diabetes.

Q.4. What are the complications of gestational diabetes?

Ans. Diabetes can affect the developing baby throughout the pregnancy. In early pregnancy, a mother's diabetes can result in birth defects and an increased rate of miscarriage. Many of the birth defects that occur. Affect major organs such as the brain and heart.

During the second and third trimester, a mother's diabetes can lead to overnutrition and excess growth of the baby. Having a large baby increases risks during labor and delivery.

For example, large babies often require cesarean deliveries and if he or she is delivered vaginally, they are at increased risk for trauma to their shoulder.

In addition, when fetal overnutrition occurs and hyper insulinemia results, the baby's blood sugar can drop very low after birth, since it will not be receiving the high blood sugar from the mother. However, with proper treatment, we can deliver a healthy baby despite having diabetes.

Q.5. Who is at risk for gestational diabetes?

Ans. The following factors increase the risk of developing gestational diabetes during pregnancy:

- Being overweight prior to becoming pregnant (if you are 20% or more over ideal body weight)
- Being a member of a high-risk ethnic group (Hispanic, Black, Native American, or Asian)
- Having sugar in urine
- Impaired glucose tolerance or impaired fasting glucose (blood sugar levels are high, but not high enough to be diabetes)
- Family history of diabetes (if parents or siblings have diabetes)
- Previously giving birth to a baby over 9 pounds
- Previously giving birth to a stillborn baby
- Having gestational diabetes with a previous pregnancy
- Having too much amniotic fluid (a condition called polyhydramnios)

Many women who develop gestational diabetes have no known risk factors.

Q.6. What are the symptoms of diabetes during pregnancy?

Ans. Symptoms of diabetes during pregnancy are:

- Increased thirst
- **Need to urinate more often:** One indicator of pregnancy is the increased need to urinate. Normally, it occurs between 6 to 8 weeks after conception

- **Fatigue:** Pregnancy signs of tiredness are very common. Slowing down a bit might help. Body is just exhausted from all the regular tasks like running
- **Nausea and vomiting:** It can happen immediately, at the beginning of pregnancy. Vomiting can occur at morning, noon or night. It will usually happen in the first trimester of pregnancy and end by the second trimester. Some women will continue this morning sickness with it until giving birth
- **Increased thirst and hunger:** Although patient may feel hungry, she may lose weight. If patient begin becoming thinner may be because of continuous sick
- **Frequent infections:** Including those of the bladder, vagina, and skin might be a symptom of diabetes
- The vision is often blurry.

CHAPTER 22

Infertility

Q.1. What is Infertility?

Ans. If a woman after marriage, with unprotected intercourse does not become pregnant she is called infertile.

Q.2. Is it related to age of the woman?

Ans. Yes, the woman is most fertile between ages of 18–24 (60–80%). The fertility goes down as age advances and becomes as low as 5–10% after the age of 40.

Q.3. What are the causes of female infertility?

Ans. Causes of female infertility are:

Female infertility may occur when:

- Autoimmune disorders, such as antiphospholipid syndrome (APS)
- Cancer or tumor
- Clotting disorders
- Growths (such as fibroids or polyps) in the uterus and cervix
- Birth defects that affect the reproductive tract
- Excessive exercising
- Eating disorders or poor nutrition
- Use of certain medications, including chemotherapy drugs
- Obesity, older age
- Ovarian cysts and polycystic ovary syndrome (PCOS)
- Pelvic infection or pelvic inflammatory disease (PID)
- Scarring from sexually transmitted infection or endometriosis.

Causes of Failure to Ovulate

- **Hormonal problems:** Any hormonal disruption can hinder ovulation. There are three main sources causing this problem:
  - Failure to produce mature eggs.
  - Malfunction of the hypothalamus.
  - Malfunction of the pituitary gland.
- **Scarred ovaries:** Physical damage to the ovaries for example, extensive, invasive, or multiple surgeries, Infection.
- **Follicle problems:** "unruptured follicle syndrome".
- Causes of poorly functioning fallopian tubes

  - **Infection:** Example is hydrosalpnix
  - Abdominal Diseases: Appendicitis and colitis, causing inflammation of the abdominal cavity
  - Ectopic pregnancy
- Endometriosis
- **Additional factors:** Fibroid, polyps and adenomyosis
- Congenital abnormalities, such as septate uterus
- Behavioral Factors:
  - Diet and exercise
  - Personal habits and lifestyle factors
  - Smoking, alcohol
  - **Drug:** Drugs, such as marijuana and anabolic steroids, cocaine.

Environmental and occupational factors: Exposure to various toxins or chemicals in the workplace or the surrounding

Q. 4. What are the causes of male infertility?

Ans. Male infertility can be caused by:
- **Smoking:** Significantly decreases both sperm count and sperm cell motility
- Prolonged use of marijuana and other recreational drugs
- Chronic alcohol abuse
- **Anabolic steroid use:** Causes testicular shrinkage and infertility
- Overly intense exercise: Produces high levels of adrenal steroid hormones
- Inadequate vitamin C, D and Zinc in the diet
- Tight underwear: Increases scrotal temperature which results in decreased sperm production
- Exposure to environmental hazards and toxins such as pesticides, lead, paint, radiation, radioactive substances, mercury, benzene, boron, and heavy metals
- Malnutrition and anemia
- Excessive stress
- Injuries or other damage to the reproductive system
- Sperm that do not work properly
- Anatomical problems: Sperm abnormalities, birth defects
- Disease, chemical exposure, and lifestyle habits
- Abnormal sperm morphology structural abnormalities, cryptorchidism, Hypospadias
- Hormonal deficiencies: Hypogonadism
- Genetic disorders—Cystic fibrosis, Polycystic kidney disease, Klinefelter syndrome, Kartagener syndrome
- Being in high heat for prolonged periods
- Impotence, Infection, older age
- Cancer treatments, including chemotherapy and radiation
- Retrograde ejaculation

Use of certain drugs, suchas cimetidine, spironolactone, and nitrofurantoin.

Q.5. Is it related to time period after marriage?

Ans. Just after the marriage, due to more frequency of intercourse, chance of pregnancy is more. More the years of marriage the couple has more unexplained infertility.

Q.6. When should the couple see the infertility specialist?

Ans. After marriage, if the couple is unable to get pregnancy within one year of their expecting it, they should see the infertility doctor immediately and should not waste time.

Q.7. What is superovulation?

Ans. In this treatment medicines like clomiphene citrate, letrozole and hormonal injections of FSH and LH or recombinant FSH are given daily to get more than one follicle which then is made to rupture by giving injection of HCG. This process increases chances of pregnancy by 30–40%. The risk of multiple pregnancy and ovarian hyperstimulation syndrome (OHSS) is there, so this is to be done judiciously.

Q.8. What investigations does a couple have to undergo in infertility work-up?

Ans. Routine investigations include blood counts including HIV and HbsAG in both partners.

- Tests for checking tubal patency– HSG, SSG
- HSG–Hysterosalpingography: In this, a radiopaque dye is injected inside the uterus and X–ray is taken to see the tubes and uterus.
- SSG–Sonosalphigography saline is injected into the tubes and checked by 3D color doppler ultrasound machine.
- Tests for ovulation
  - **BBT:** Basal body temperature chart, urinary LH, serum progesterone on 21st day of the menses, ultrasound follicular monitoring, and endometrial biopsy on 2nd day of the menses to see the ovulation.
- Special Investigation
  - Hormone assays: On 2nd day of the menses— FSH, LH, E2 (estradiol) serum Prolactin, TSH
  - Videoendoscopy
  - Hysterolaparoscopy: In this, we inspect uterus, tubes ovaries and tubal patency with the help of endoscopes
  - Transvaginal ultrasonography.

Q.9. What is diagnostic hysterosaparoscopy (Video endoscopy)? Is it necessary in all cases?

Ans. Diagnostic and SOS therapeutic hysterosaparoscopy is a small operation (Procedure) done under anesthesia (CA). It is a day care procedure and patients are discharged on the same day. In this operation a laparoscope is introduced. In the abdomen the uterus, tubes, ovaries, pouch of douglas and bowel is visualized. Tubal potency is confirmed by injection of dye. Small corrective operations are also done through laparoscope such as ovarian drilling, adhesionolysis excision of myomas, endometriomas, cauterization, etc. Through hysteroscope the uterine cavity is visualized. Polyps, fibroids, septum, etc. is diagnosed and treated. Tubal osteas can be visualized and can be treated if necessary. At the end of a hysteroslaparoscopy the diagnosis of infertility is definitely established and a treatment plan is made. It is better to do a hysteroslaparoscopy in all cases of infertility before strong treatment. However it may be differed or delayed in some cases such as:

- Young patients just married with no obvious disease who may be given trial by direct treatment cycle
- Cost Consideration: If patient refuses to spend for it then alternative methods of determining tubal potency such as HSG or sonosalpingography may be performed
- If patient has undergone laparoscopy earlier
- If patient is unfit to undergo operation

A good diagnostic hysteroslaparoscopy is the gold standard basic investigation in infertility work-up.

Q.10. Is it necessary to get all these investigations done and spend so much money?

Ans. A good work–up at a good centre pays in the long run; results will come faster and cheaper in the long run. Incomplete work-up will result in halfhearted treatment which will delay pregnancy and total cost will go up.

Q.11. What are the usual treatment options given to the patient?

Ans. Usually during a hysterolaparoscopy, undergoing problems are diagnosed and treated. The following treatment options are available to the patient:

- Planned Relations
- Super ovulation with intra uterine insemination. In super ovulation with IUI the woman is given hormones (oral and injectables) to stimulate her ovaries to produce more eggs. Follicular developments is monitored using serial ultra-sonography when the follicles are mature, a hormonal injection is given to help them rupture. Then an intrauterine insemination is done using washed capacitated sperms. If the sperm count is good then this procedure has a 40–50% success rate and the patient has a good chance of getting pregnant in 3 cycles.

Q.12. What is IVF–ET (In Vitro Fertilization Embryo Transfer) Test–Tube baby? When is this needed to be done?

Ans. IVF–ET is needed to be done is patients with blocked fallopian tubes. It may also be done in other forms of infertility where IUI superovulation has failed. In this the woman is subjected to controlled ovarian hyperstimulation using hormonal injections. Many more injection are required because we want to retrieve as many eggs as possible. Once the follicles have reached an appropriate size, vaginal ovum aspiration is done and the ova are collected in a petridish with a media. Capacitated sperms are then mixed with oocytes and fertilization is achieved into the uterus. Once embryos are formed then they (2–3 embryos) are transferred into the uterus on day 3 or day 5. Progesterone support is then given chemical pregnancy is diagnosed by B–HCG on day 30. Live pregnancy is confirmed by 5 weeks by seeing a live fetal heart on vaginal sonography.

Q.13. What is assisted reproductive technology (ART)?

Ans. Assisted reproductive technology (ART) is a group of different methods used to help infertile couples. ART works by removing eggs from a woman's body. The eggs are then mixed with sperm to make embryos. The embryos are then put back in the woman's body.

Q.14. What are the success rates of ART?

Ans. Success rates on ART for some fertility clinics. According to the 2006 CDC report on ART, the average percentage of ART cycles that led to a live birth were:

- 39% in women under the age of 35
- 30% in women aged 35–37
- 21% in women aged 37–40
- 11% in women aged 41–42

ART can be expensive and time-consuming. But it has allowed many couples to have children that otherwise would not have been conceived.

Q.15. What are the common complication of ART?

Ans. The most common complication of ART is multiple fetuses. But this is a problem that can be prevented or minimized in several different ways.

Q.16. How often is assisted reproductive technology (ART) successful?

Ans. Success rates vary and depend on many factors. Somethings that affect the success rate of ART include:

- Age of the partners
- Reason for infertility
- Clinic
- Type of art
- If the egg is fresh or frozen
- If the embryo is fresh or frozen.

Q.17. What is ICSI and when is it done?

Ans. ICSI is Intra Cytoplasmic Sperm Injection. In this, a single sperm is injected into the oocyte using an robotic micro manipulator. Other steps are same as IVF.

Q.18. What are the indication of intracytoplasmic sperm injection?

Ans. Indication of ICSI include:

a. Severe Oligospermia
b. Azospermia where sperms are retrieved from epididymis or test
c. Failed fertilization in IVF

In fact ICSI has revolutionized treatment of male factor infertility.

Q.19. What are the other options for patients with nil sperms or very low count of sperms?

Ans. The other options apart from ICSI are:

a. Donor insemination
b. Adoption

Donor may be brought by the patient (relative, friend, etc.) or may be from sperm bank. Many case of donor sperm donor must be screened for VDRL, HIV, HbsAg, genetic disorders, blood group, caste, educational status, built color of skin, hair, eyes and any other specific features are also taken into consideration.

Q.20. What is operative endoscopy? How does it help in infertility?

Ans. With advance technology, minimal invasive method can be used to remove different obstructions in the way of woman's fertility.

- With operative hysteroscopy: Septum, fibroid and polyps and adhesions (synuchiae) inside uterus can be removed. Cornual catheterization can open the proximal tubal block

- Operative Laparoscopy: Along with checking the uterus, tubes and ovaries it can treat the diseases like, fibroids, endometriosis, ovarian cysts, dermiod, polycystic ovaries, adhesions and also do tubal microsurgery.

Q.21. What are the prevention should be taken for infertility?

Ans. Prevention should be taken are:

- Preventing sexually transmitted infections (STIs), such as gonorrhea and chlamydia, may reduce risk of infertility
- Maintaining a healthy diet, weight, and lifestyle may increase chances for getting pregnant and having a healthy pregnancy
- Take a prenatal or multivitamin containing folate before and during pregnancy. This lowers risk for miscarriage and developmental problems in the baby.

Q.22. What are the steps required to get pregnant?

Ans. Pregnancy is the result of a process that has many steps

To get pregnant:

- A woman must release an egg from one of her ovaries (ovulation)
- The egg must go through a fallopian tube toward the uterus (womb)
- A man's sperm must join with (fertilize) the egg along the way
- The fertilized egg must attach to the inside of the uterus (implantation)

Infertility can happen if there are problems with any of these steps.

Q.23. What is Hysterosalpingogram?

Ans. Hysterosalpingogram is procedure shows some of the internal anatomy of the tubes. If tubal surgery is planned it is an important additional test as grading of tubal pathology can give some prognostic information about the outcome of the surgery.

Q.24. How laparoscopy help in treating infertility?

Ans. Laparoscopy aids the diagnosis of uterine and tubal problems as it allows direct vision of the exterior of the uterus and tubes. It requires general anesthesia and involves a minimum of two small cuts (approx 1 cm long) in the abdomen, usually one in the region of the navel (umbilicus) and the other in the pelvic region. This direct form of looking at the uterus and tubes is useful in the diagnosis of blocked or scarred tubes, and also in examining the relationship of the tube to the ovary. The injection of a coloured dye through the cervix and observing it filling and spilling from the fallopian tubes is a good test of wether or not the tubes are blocked or not.

The doctor can assess the state of health of the fingerlike processes at the end of the tube (fimbriae), which are vitally important for egg collection. Various degrees of corrective surgery can be performed at the same time and these involve making additional small holes in the abdomen. Finally, the remainder of the pelvis may be examined to exclude conditions such as endometriosis, as well as other organs in the abdominal cavity. Laparoscopy normally requires a hospital stay of a few hours to one day.

Key Terms

- **Breech presentation:** The condition in which the baby enters the birth canal with its buttocks or feet first

- **Cephalopelvic disproportion:** The condition in which the babys head is too large to fit through the mother's pelvis
- **Cervical Circlage:** It is a procedure in which sutures are used to close the cervix, the lower part of the uterus that opens to the vagina during pregnancy to help prevent premature birth. It is a treatment for cervical incompetence.
- **Doula:** A doula is someone who undergoes special training to enable them to support women during childbirth and into the postpartum period
- **Dystocia:** Failure to progress in labor, either because the cervix will not dilate (expand) further or because the head does not descend through the mother's pelvis after full dilation of the cervix
- **Genital herpes:** A life–long, recurrent sexually transmitted infection caused by the herpes simplex virus (HSV)
- **Perinatal:** Referring to the period of time surrounding an infants birth, from the last two months of pregnancy through the first 28 days of life
- **Pitocin:** A synthetic hormone that produces uterine contractions
- Placenta previa: A condition in which the placenta totally or partially covers the cervix, preventing vaginal delivery
- **Placental abruption:** A abnormal separation of the placenta from the uterus before the birth of the baby, with subsequent heavy uterine bleeding. Normally, the baby is born first and then the placenta is delivered within a half hour
- Postpartal: The six-week period following childbirth
- **Rh blood incompatibility:** Incompatibility between the blood of a mother and her baby due the absence of the Rh antigen in the red blood cells of one and its presence in the red blood cells of the other
- **Umbilical cord prolapse:** A birth situation in which the umbilical cord, the structure that connects the placenta to the umbilicus of the fetus to deliver oxygen and nutrients, falls out of the uterus and becomes compressed, thus preventing the delivery of oxygen.

SECTION 2

Psychiatric Nursing

- Introduction of Mental Health Nursing
- Community Mental Health Nursing
- Description of Terminology Based on Disorder of Thinking, Mood Perception and Memory
- Review of Personality and Defense Mechanism
- Disorder of Perception Schizophrenia
- Disorder of Mood and Affect
- Anxiety Disorder
- Substance Abuse and Alcoholism
- Eating and Personality Disorder
- Mental Retardation
- Organic Brain Disorder
- Psychiatric Emergency
- Psychotherapeutic Modalities

CHAPTER

23

Introduction of Mental Health Nursing

Q.1. Who explained brain pathology first?

Ans. The Hippocrates (460 BC) a Greek physician is known as father of Modern Medicine, explain brain pathology as mental illness and classified as mania melancholia and phrenitis. He recommended marriage as a treatment for mental illness.

Q.2. Who is founder of psychology?

Ans. Sigmund reud is the father of psychology who had given theory of psychoanalysis.

Q.3. Who is first psychiatry nurse?

Ans. Linda Richards is first American Psychiatry nurse graduated from New England Hospital.

Q.4. Who explained interpersonal theory of psychiatry nursing?

Ans. Hildegard Peplau mother of psychiatry nursing has explained interpersonal theory of therapeutic relationship in nursing practice.

Q.5. Which year doctoral programme started?

Ans. In 1960 in Boston first doctoral programme for psychiatry nursing was started in the same year first mental health year was celebrated.

Q.6. Where was the first Indian mental hospital constructed?

Ans. First Indian Mental Hospital was constructed at Calcutta.

Q.7. In which year Lunancy Act founded?

Ans. First Lunancy Act was amended by British parliament by 1858.

Q.8. When term 'asylum' was replaced by term hospital?

Ans. The term asylum was replaced by hospital in 1920.

Q.9. Who introduced "Therapeutic Community"?

Ans. Maxwell Jone's in 1953 defined concept of therapeutic community.

Q.10. When was the first community mental health centre was established?

Ans. The first community mental health centre was established in Raipur Rani Block of Ambala district in Haryana State.

Q.11. What is Mental Health Act?

Ans. Mental Health Act is a bill for safety protection of legal rights of mentally ill client, provided by Indian Constitution. It was sanctioned in 1987, 22nd May by Indian Parliament.

Q.12. What are the admission criteria for psychiatry patient?

Ans. Admission of psychiatry patient can be done under following terms and basis:

a. On voluntary basis by client or nearest guardian

b. Admission of mentally ill prisoners may be admitted into mental hospital on the order of presiding officer or a court

c. Admission under certain special circumstances through relatives or friends

d. Admission through magistrate of the area and by police officer

e. Admission in emergency if patient is dangerous for others.

Q.13. Who is responsible to give discharge sheet to psychiatry clients?

Ans. The medical officer in charge of psychiatric hospital or psychiatric nursing home on recommendation of other psychiatrist by order in writing direct the discharge of mentally ill patient.

Q.14. What is law of marriage of a lunatic person?

Ans. According to Hindu Marriage Act of 1955 under section 12 of A marriage with a person who was an idiot or lunatic can be declared null in this case either party to a marriage may present an application for judicial separation.

Q.15. What is law for adoption for a mentally ill patient?

Ans. **a.** Act 78 (1965) section: 7 provided law of adoption that is a Hindu male 'who is of sound mind is not' the consent of his wife unless- she has been declared by a court to be of unsound mind

b. A Hindu female 'who is of sound mind' is not a minor and is not married can adopt a child. If she is married and her husband has been declared by court to be of unsound mind (under section 8).

Q.16. What is Narcotic Drug and Psychotropic Substances Act?

Ans. In 1985 NDPSA declared if any person produces, possesses, transports, imports, exports drugs or psychotropic substance except 'Ganja' he shall be punishable with

I. Rigorous imprisonment for not less than 2 years which may extend to 20 years and

II. A fine not less that 1 lakh rupees which may extend to 2 lakh rupees

III. Punishment for repeat offence is RI for not less than 15 years which may extend to 30 years and a fine of not less than 1.5 lakh to 3 lakh rupees.

Q.17. What are protections of human rights of mentally ill person provided by IMHA?

Ans. Under section 81 of Indian Mental Health Act 1987:

1. No mentally ill person shall be subjected during treatment to any indignity (Physical/Mental) or cruelty.
2. No mentatly ill person under treatment shall be used for purpose of research unless:
   - **a.** It is directly benefited to him (diagnostically and treatment wise)
   - **b.** Research can be done only after valid consent of voluntary or by guardian.

Q.18. What are rights of mentally ill patient by IMHA?

Ans
1. The right to wear their own cloths
2. Right to keep and use their own personal possessions

3. Right to keep and be allowed to spend a reasonable sum of their money for canteen expenses and small purchases
4. Right to keep individual storage
5. Right to see visitors everyday
6. Right to make and receive calls and access letter writing materials
7. Right to refuse electroconvulsive therapy
8. Right to manage and dispose of property
9. Right to execute wills
10. Right to hold civil service status.

Q.19. What are the legal roles of psychiatry nurse?

Ans.
1. Nurse should aware of Indian Mental Health Act.
2. She should be qualified to work in a psychiatric ward or go through a continuing education program.
3. She should be aware of procedure of admission and discharge.
4. In the case of leave/absence or abscond, she should informed to concerned psychiatrist or police office.
5. She should be aware of rights of mentally ill patient.
6. Should obtain informed consent for treatment and procedure. (All therapy like ECT).
7. Maintenance of confidentiality of records and record keeping.
8. Maintain the standards of nursing care.

Q.20. What is mental health team?

Ans.
1. Teamwork is more significant in a mental health setting where contribution of all members is vital for assessment diagnosis treatment and rehabilitation purpose. Members of the mental health team:
2. Psychiatrist
3. Psychiatric nurse clinical specialist
4. Registered nurse working in a psychiatric unit
5. Clinical psychologist
6. Psychiatric social worker
7. Psychiatric para-professionals
8. Psychiatric Aids – ECT Technician
9. Occupational therapist
10. Diversional/Play therapist
11. Creative art therapist
12. Clergy man.

Q.21. What is mental health? Define it.

Ans. Mental health is an integral part of total health of an individual. According to meninger, "Mental Health is the adjustment of human being to each other and to the world around them with a maximum of effectiveness and happiness" Mental health is an individual and personal matter.

Q.22. What are the criteria of positive mental health?

Ans. Jahoda has describe six criteria for positive mental health are as follows:

1. Positive attitude towards self in relation to self-awareness, confidence, self-esteem and sense of identification towards, role, social norms, strength and weakness
2. Growth, development and self-actualization means individual must seek for new growth, new development and new challenges
3. **Integration:** Integration means capacity of an individual to maintain balance between Id, ego and superego
4. **Autonomy:** Autonomy is ability to regulate individual's decision making and action
5. **Perception of reality:** A mentally healthy people is able to change his perception in the light of new information
6. **Environmental Mastery:** It is ability to adapt adjust and behave appropriately according with situation with sociocultural norms.

Q.23. What are the classification systems used to classify mental disorder?

Ans. Major classification of mental disorder are:

1. International Classification of Disease (ICD X)
2. Diagnostic Statistical Manual classification (DSM–III R)
3. Research Diagnostic Criteria (RDC)

These classification permit mental health workers to compare, incidence, types of disorders and relevant data concerning mental disorders throughout the world

ICD X: In ICD X code numbers has given to left hand side for example:

F00-F09: Organic symptomatic, mental disorder

F10–F10: Alcohol and drug abuse disorder

- Dementia
- Delirium
- Amnestic syndrome
- F20–F29: schizophrenia, schizotypal and delusional disorder.

In DSM IV Revised classification system

Diseases are classify on various axes

Axis I – Clinical symptoms

Axis II – Personality disorder

Axis III – Physical disorders

Axis IV – Severity of psychosocial stressors like death of close one.

Axis V – Highest level of adaptive functioning in the post year.

ICDX is more descriptive whereas DSM and RDC are for research purpose only.

In DSM diagnosis is based on presence of symptoms in active phase for (4 symptoms) at least one to four week of duration like delusion hallucination loosening of association, catatonic behavior inappropriate effect, etc. for diagnosing a case of schizophrenia.

According to RDC atleast two of the following symptoms for diagnosis schizophrenia are essential.

Withdrawal, delusion, persecution, hallucination, period of illness lasting 2 weeks.

Q.24. Define primary cause, predisposing cause and precipitatory cause of mental illness.

Ans. **Primary cause:** primary cause means it is the condition without which the disorder would not have occurred for example, in head injury trauma lead to confusional state, that is a primary cause

Predisposing cause: It is the condition that comes before the disease has occurred or psychopathology has appeared, e.g. Rejection by parents in the early age of child will cause disease of later age of 16 to 18 or 30 to 40 years like personality disorder, drug abuse anxiety disorder, etc.

Precipitatory cause: It is a condition that becomes too much for an individual to tolerate and triggers to maladaptive behavior, e.g. death of the father of an adolescent boy may lead him into depression.

Q.25. What are the causes of mental illness?

Ans. Cause of mental illness are as follows:

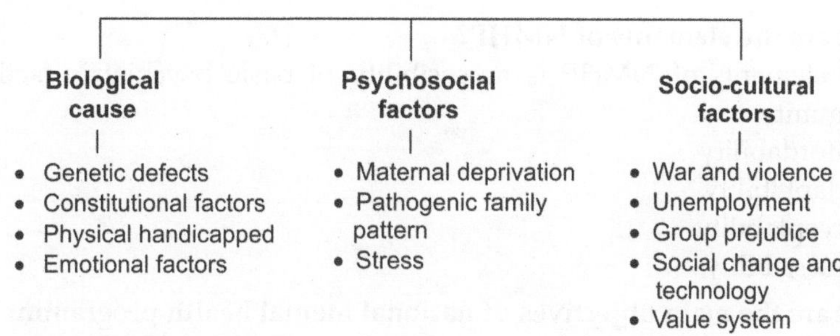

CHAPTER 24

Community Mental Health Nursing

Q.1. What are the elements of NMHP?

Ans. Basic elements of NMHP is accessibility of basic psychiatric facilities within community.

- Affordability
- Adaptability
- Acceptability
- Assessibility

Q.2. What are the main objectives of national mental health programme?

Ans. The objectives are following:

1. To ensure availability and accessibility of minimum mental health care for all
2. To encourage application of mental health knowledge in general health care
3. To promote community participation in the mental health service.

Q.3. What are the levels of prevention in psychiatry?

Ans. There are three level of prevention in psychiatry

1. Primary prevention
2. Secondary prevention
3. Tertiary prevention.

Q.4. What are the nurses role in primary prevention?

Ans. Role of nurse in primary prevention is:

1. Providing skilled antenatal care and educating the mother regarding the adverse effects of irradiation; drugs and irradiation
2. Prevent effect of anoxia and Injury to newborn at birth
3. Providing dietary correction for the metabolic disorder
4. Correcting endocrinal disorders
5. Providing training program for mentally and physically handicapped children
6. Counselling for people for adaptive coping techniques
7. Extending mental health education services at general level.

Q.5. What are nurse role in secondary level of prevention?

Ans. Role of nurse in secondary level of prevention is as follows:

1. Assisting in early diagnostic and case finding
2. Early referral of sensitive cases

3. Screening program for adolescent, ANC and other psychological deprived people
4. Providing early and effective treatment
5. Providing mental health education to general people
6. Assisting in crisis intervention
7. Providing short term counselling and consultation services.

Q. 6. What are the nurses role in tertiary prevention?

Ans. Main role of nurses in tertiary level of prevention are:

1. Social reintegration of the discharged and chronic mentally ill back into the community
2. Vocational rehabilitation and job placement for the mentally retarded
3. Teach and trained skill training and activity of daily living to mentally ill patient
4. Utilizing the resources of family and community for the long term rehabilitation.

CHAPTER

25 Description of Terminology Based on Disorder of Thinking, Mood Perception and Memory

Q.1. What are the disorder of perception?

Ans. Perception is sensory feeling to any internal or external stimuli. The abnormality or disorder of perception are as below:

1. **Illusion:** It is miss-perception of external stimuli, e.g. a person on a dark night can miss perceive a rope as a snake
2. **Hallucination:** It is a perception experienced in the absence of external stimuli to the sense organs. The types of hallucination depends on the sensory systems affected, e.g. Auditory, visual, olfactory, gustatory and tactile.

Q.2. What are the types of hallucination?

Ans. Types of hallucination are:

1. **Auditory hallucination:** Auditory hallucination may be experienced as noises, music or voices, patient experience commentary voices or noises usually which is vague not clear. This is common in schizophrenia
2. **Visual hallucinations:** It may be experienced as seeing person, objects, or animals the size may be normal or abnormal. This is also common in schizophrenia and psychotic disorder
3. **Olfactory hallucination:** Olfactory hallucinations experienced as unpleasant smells
4. **Gustatory hallucination:** This is experience as unpleasant tastes in mouth patient think that somebody is added bitter taste in food. This is rare but occur in schizophrenia and in sever depression.

Tactile hallucination: Tactile hallucination are experienced as sensation of being touched, pricked or strangled by insects or worm, etc. this usually occur in person who abuse alcohol, cocaine, etc. rarely experienced by schizophrenic client.

Q.3. Define thinking process. What are the abnormal thoughts in psychiatry client?

Ans. **Thinking:** Thinking is ideational and informational component of mental activity. Thinking occurs through manipulation of verbal and nonverbal symbol images, music and kin esthetic sensation

Abnormal thoughts are:

- **Retarted thinking:** Retarded thinking means speed of thought is slowed down
- **Thought blocking:** In thoughts block there is sudden break in train of thoughts patient feels his mind has gone blank: observer notices a sudden interruption in the patient's speech.

- **Pressure of thought:** In pressure of thought ideas arise in unusual variety and abundance and pass through the mind rapidly.
- **Poverty of thought:** In poverty of thought the patient has few thoughts and these lack variety and richness and seems to move slowly through the minds

Disorder of the form of thought
(Linking of thoughts together)

- **Flight of ideas:** In flight of ideas the thoughts and speech move quickly from one topic to another.
- **Clang association:** A second word with a sound similar to the first
- **Punning:** A second meaning of the first word.
- **Circumstantialities:** In circumstantialities there is slowed thinking patient reached finally goal after so many trivial details.
- **Tangentially:** In tangentially patient follows a series of related topics but never reaches to the goal.
- **Loosening of association:** Loosening of association often mirrors the client's artistic thoughts and reflects the person's poorly organized thinking, e.g. word salad and verbigeration that is senseless repetition of words and phrases where one thought can not match to another.
- **Magical thinking:** In magical thinking there is belief that specific action thought posturing will fulfill certain wishes and word of certain evils.

Q.4. What is Delusion?

Ans.
- **Abnormal thought content delusion:** A delusions is a false unshakable belief that cannot be changed by others there are various forms of delusion.
  - **Primary Delusion:** A primary delusion is one that appears suddenly and with full conviction but without any mental events leading up to it.
  - **Secondary delusions:** Secondary delusion is derived from a pervious morbid experience.
  - **Delusion persecution:** In persecutory delusion patient believes that person or organization are trying to inflict harm on the patient, damage his reputation properly or make him insane or poison him these are seen in organic psychosis and in paranoid schizophrenia.
  - **Delusion of reference:** Person believes that objects events or people have personal significance for the patient, e.g. words on newspaper or in Radio are believed to be directed to the patient this is also seen in paranoid schizophrenia.
  - **Grandiose delusions:** Are beliefs of exaggerated self-importance the patient may think he is a multimillionaire a king or prime minister of country, etc. Mainly seen in mania and schizophrenia.
  - **Delusion of guilt and worthlessness:** It is often seen in depression in this client have rependation of every mistake and fault with him/herself only he or she blame self for every unfortunate.
  - **Nihilistic delusions:** It is seen is severe depression patient feels that body parts are missing or there is failure of bodily function.
  - **Hypochondriacally delusions:** This is seen in somatic disorder contrary to medical evidence the patient may believe wrongly that he is ill.

- **Delusion of Jealousy:** Seen usually in males the individual is obsessed with doubts about the spouses fidelity is seen commonly in paranoid states it is also called delusion of infidelity.
- **Delusion of control:** The patient believes that his action, impulses or thought are controlled by an outside agency. This is also seen in schizophrenia.

- **Other abnormal thoughts at content level are:**
  - **Preoccupation:** In preoccupation the patient continuously reflects on one topic or a group of topics to the exclusion of environmental late rests and to the detriment of useful activity. This may seen in schizophrenia anxiety disorder obsessive compulsive disorder.
- **Obsession:** Obsessions is persistent and recurrent thoughts, impulses or images that enter the mind without wish of patient.
- **Over valued ideas:** Over valued idea is a false or unreasonable belief that is sustained beyond the bound of reason.

Q.5. What is abnormal thoughts possession?

Ans. Abnormal thoughts possession are:

- **Thoughts insertion:** The patient believes that certain thoughts are not the patients own but inserted into his mind by an outside agency.
- **Thoughts broad casting:** Patient believes that other people can hear or come to know their thoughts.
- **Thoughts withdrawal:** The patient believes that other people or forces are removing thoughts from the patient mind.

Q. 6. Define mood and affect?

Ans. **Mood:** Mood is pervasive and sustained emotion that (internal emotional feeling) that colors the perception of the world, e.g. happy mood cheerful, sad mood, anxious mood, etc.

Affect: Affect is a pattern of observable behavior (expression of emotion), e.g. sadness, elation and anger.

Q.7. What are the disorder or abnormal mood?

Ans. **Disorder of mood are following:** (4 E of Mood)

Euphoria: It is mild elevation of mood in which increased sense of psychological well-being and happiness not in keeping with the ongoing events seen in hypomania.

Elation: It moderate elevation of mood in this feeling of confidence and enjoyment along with increased psychomotor activity this is seen in mania stage – II

Exaltation: It is severe elevation of mood in this intense elation with of illusion of grandeur seen in severe mania stage – III.

Ecstasy: It is very severe elevation of mood, it is sense of intense sense of blissfulness even in delirious or stuporuse mania stage – IV.

Euthymia: It is normal range of mood with absence of depressed or elevated mood.

Dysphoria: Dysphoria is an unpleased mood, such as anxiety, sadness or irritability.

Irritable mood: Easily annoyed and provoked to anger.

Alexithymia: Difficulty in being aware of or describing one's emotion.

Mood Swing: It is emotional feeling between period of elation and depression.

Apathy: Loss of emotional tone and ability to feel pleasure

Depressed mood: A feeling of sadness loneliness, despair low self esteem and crying spells.

Disorder of Affect:

Restricted/Constricted affect: Mild reduction in the range and intensity of emotional expression.

Blunted affect: Severe reduction in the intensity of emotional expresson

Flat affect: Absence of any affective expression

Inappropriate affect: Discordance between affective expression and content of speech

Labile affect: Affective expression characterized by repeated rapid and abrupt shifts cannot related to external stimuli

Incongruous affect: Laughs, giggles or smiles without eye contact patient may cry or wail when contest of speech is neutral or even pleasant.

Q.8. Define the following words:

Ans. **a.** Palilalia: The patient repeats a word with increasing frequency

b. Logo lonia: In this patient repeats a word the last syllable of last word

c. Echopraxia: Echophraxia the patient imitates action they see patient do it so when not asked to do

d. Echolalia: In echolalia there is automatic imitation by patient of another person's speech. It is repetitive and persistent.

Q.9. Differentiate the term catalepsy and cataplexy.

Ans. **Catalepsy (Waxy flexibility):** Catalepsy is a condition in which person maintain abnormal or uncomfortable position for long periods observed in severe cases of catatonic schizophrenia.

Cataplexy: Cataplexy describes a temporary sudden locks of muscle, causing weakness and immobilization can be precipitated by a variety of emotional states and is often following by sleep this is commonly seen in narcolepsy.

Q.10. Give one word answer:

Ans.

1. Partial or total inability to recall past experiences is called Amnesia
2. Loss of memory of events that occur after the onset of etiological condition **Anterogradeamnesia**
3. Loss of memory of past events and not progressive **Retrograde amnesia**
4. An exaggerated degree of retention and recall of memory is called as **Hypermnesia**
5. It is falsification and distortion of memory is known as **paramnesia**
6. The condition in which gaps in the memory are unconsciousnessly filled with false memories (stories farming seen in korsakoff's syndrome) called **confabulation**
7. When patient strongly feels that the current situation has been seen or experienced before is termed as **Deja uv**

Q.11. What is insight. What are the levels of insight?

Ans. Insight is degree of awareness of one's own mental condition or understanding about self-illness it has six level -

1. **Grade I:** Complete denial of illness
2. **Grade II:** Slight awareness of being sick needling help but denying it at the some time
3. **Grade III:** (Partial insight) Awareness of being sick but blaming to external factor
4. **Grade IV:** Partial insight: Awareness that of illness is present but reason is unknown
5. **Intellectual insight:** Awareness that illness is due to irrational feeling disturbance
6. **True emotional insight:** (Full insight) when patient awareness of their own mental condition and needing and seeking medical advice and also wish to change in their behavior or personality.

Q.12. How do you assess level of judgment?

Ans. Judgment is the ability to choose appropriate goal and to select socially acceptable and appropriate means to reach them. It reflect reality testing intelligence and experience. It is tested by giving or asking some reality situation to patient and their response in same way.

Judgment: Judgment is rated on Good/Intact/Normal

Social Judgment: Social judgment is observed during the hospital stay and during the interview session it one include personal judgment in which patient can verbilize their view of his potential limit, e.g. How does the future look to you.

Test Judgment: It is tested by asking some situation like if a house on fire (what he would do) or a man lying on road, etc.

Q.13. Match the following:

Ans.

A	B
• Dipsomania	A compulsion to steal object not for their intrinsic value
• Kleptomania	A compulsion to pullout one's own hair
• Trichotillomania	A compulsion to drink alcohol
13. Correct Matching	
• Dipsomania	A compulsion to drink alcohol.
• Kleptomania	A compulsion to steal object not for their intrinsic value.
• Trichotillomania	A compulsion to pullout one's own hair.

Q.14. What do you mean by disorder of self-awareness?

Ans. Disorder of self-awareness includes depersonalization and derealization.

Depersonalization: It is attention in the perception or experience of the self so that one feels detached from, and as if one is an outside observer of one's mental processes or body (e.g. feeling like one is in a dream)

Derealization: An alteration in the perception or experience of the external world so that it seems strange or unreal (e.g. people may seem unfamiliar or mechanical).

CHAPTER

26 Review of Personality and Defense Mechanism

Q.1. Define defense mechanism or mental process.

Ans. Defense mechanism or mental processes are at unconscious level they are used to reduce anxiety or resolve conflict this is method of self-protection defense mechanism are used to modifying or changing one's behavior. It is normal process of adjustment.

Q.2. What are defense mechanisms originated in different stage of development?

Ans. According to stage of personality development different defense mechanism are as follows:

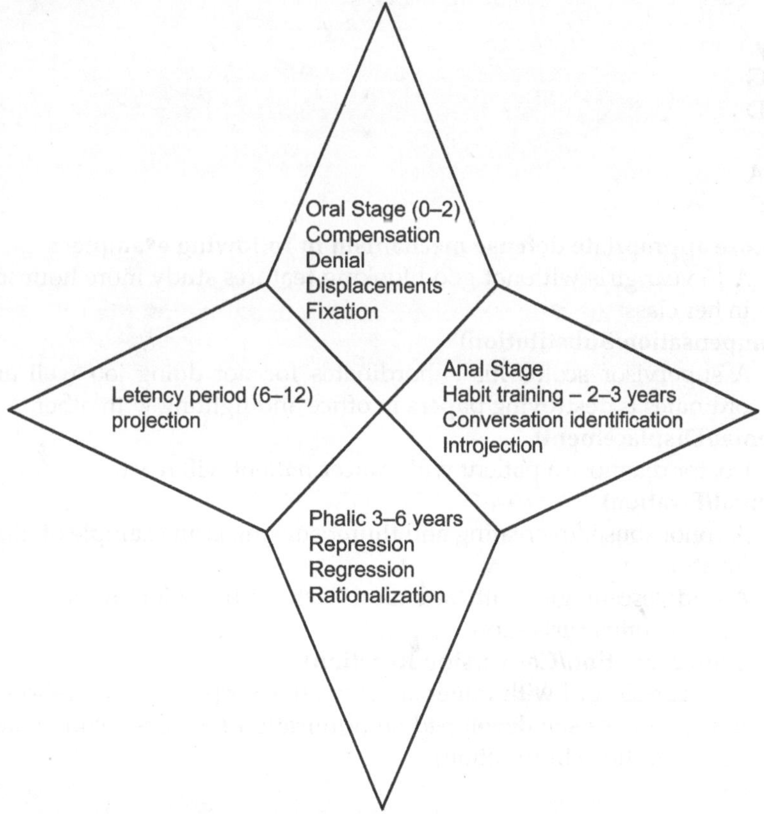

Q.3. Match appropriate defense mechanism with following column:

COLUMN A	COLUMN B
i. A process by which we inhibit the unacceptable and unwanted impulses feelings or thoughts form consciousness.	a. Rationalization
	b. Identification
	c. Sublimation
	d. Regression
ii. A process by which we avoid present difficulties by going back to an earlier less mature way of adjustment to the situation.	e. Projection
	f. Transference
	g. Repression
	h. Denial
	i. Reaction Formation
	j. Displacement
iii. Redirection of repressed impulses in to society acceptable manners.	
iv. Finding a logical reason for the things are wants to do "Sour grapes mechanism".	
v. A process in which the image of one person is unconsciously identified with that of another it may be positive or negative.	

Ans. Key

i. G
ii. D
iii. C
iv. A
v. F

Q.4. Choose appropriate defense mechanism in following example:

Ans. I. A 16 year girls with not good looking features study more hour to come first in her class:

(Compensation/Substitution)

II. A supervisor scolds his subordinates for not doing job well and the sub ordinates is destroying papers in office and fighting with other.

(Denial/Displacement)

III. Doctor diagnose a patient with cancer patient will react.

(Denial/Fixation)

IV. Alcohol abuse/overeating and thumbsucking is an example of (Substitution/ Fixation)

V. An adolescent girl with attention seeking behavior in classroom towards teachers other girls show.

(Reaction formation/Conversion Reaction)

VI. A 1-year-old girl with miner surgery after hospitalization decides to become nurse because she developed an admiration for nurse who looked after her (Identification/Introjection).

Key

i. Compensation
ii. Displacement
iii. Denial
iv. Fixation
v. Conversion
vi. Identification

Q.5. Define personality. What are the factors influencing personality?

Ans. Personality is an aggregate of the physical and mental qualities of the individual as these interact in characteristic fashion with the individual's environment.

Factor influencing personalities are:

- Heredity
- Environment and self.

Q.6. What are stages of personality development?

Ans. According to Sigmund Freud–Psychosexual development of personality development under different stages are as follows:

- Oral stage (0 to 2 years of age): During first year of life mouth is principles organ for gratification
- Anal stage (2 to 3 years): Membranes of anal region provide pleasure
- Phallic stage (3 to 6 years): Self-manipulation of genital organs
- Latency stage (6 to 12 years): It is stage of psychosexual development child involve himself/herself peer activities
- Genital stage: Final stage of psychosexual development adolescent seeking pleasure from heterosexual relation.

Q.7. Match correct personality types:

COLUMN A	COLUMN B
i. Comfort loving, pleasure seeking sentimental and socializing people soft and round people.	a. Introvort
	b. Extrovert
	c. Endomorphic
	d. Ectomorphic
	e. Morphic
ii. Very active full of energy, less religious, aggressive and noisy achievement oriented people with muscular and strong built.	f. Asthenic
iii. Sensitive delicate intellectual more religious people, with drawn prone to develop anxiety neurosis peptic ulcer very delicate and fragile.	
iv. Thin built, with drawn, occup-yed in themselves	
v. Fatty muscular people with sociable nature.	

Ans. **Key:**

i. c
ii. e
iii. d
iv. a
v. b

CHAPTER 27

Disorder of Perception Schizophrenia

Q.1. Who coined the term "Schizophrenia"

Ans. The term schizophrenia was coined in 1908 by the Swiss psychiatric Eugen Bleuler. It is derived from Greek word "Skhizo" (Split) and "Phren" (mind) meaning splitting the mind.

Q.2. Define schizophrenia.

Ans. Schizophrenia is not a simple illness "It refers to a group of mental illness characterized by specific psychological symptoms that affect the mood, regulation of emotions, thoughts, perception, emotions, movements and behavior thought process and total personality integrity"

Q.3. Which Neurochemical is responsible to develop schizophrenia?

Ans. Imbalance or dysregulation dopamine and serotonin both neurotransmitter is responsible to develop schizophrenia.

Q.4. Enlist physiological causes of schizophrenia.

Ans. Physiological causes of schizophrenia are as following:

There is high incidence of schizophrenia after:

1. Prenatal exposure to influenza virus during second trimester of pregnancy.
2. Ventricular enlargement and abnormalities of specific subregion such as amygdale, hippocampus, temporal lobes and basal ganglia in the brain.
3. Previous episodes of epilepsy.
4. Birth trauma.
5. Head injury in adulthood, alcohol abuse.
6. Huntington chorea.
7. Cerebelar tumor or CVA.
8. SLE, myxedema.
9. Parkinson's and Wilson's disease.

Q.5. What are the psychological factor which develop schizophrenia?

Ans. In psychological factor such as poor parent child relationship and dysfunctional family system causes paranoid schizophrenia.

Q.6. What are phases of development of schizophrenia?

Ans. Pattern of development of schizophrenia is viewed in four phases:

Phase I – Schizoid personality
Phase – II – Prodromal phase
Phase – III – Schizophrenia
Phase – IV – Residual phase

Phase I: In Schizoid personality individual shows very limited range of emotion he/she may be cold in emotional expression aloof and Indifferent to social relationship.

Phase II: In prodromal phase social withdrawal, impairment of role functionary, neglect hygiene and grooming, blunt or in appropriate affect, etc.

Phase III: In this active phase of schizophrenia Psychotic symptoms are prominent both positive and negative like ambivalence, associative looseness delusion hallucination and in negative symptoms alogia, anhedonia apathy blunted affect, etc. can seen along with social/occupational dysfunction.

Phase IV: In residual phase a period of remission and exacerbation is seen prognosis of illness is depend on many factors such as age, sex marital and socioeconomic status and compliance to treatment, etc.

Q.7. What are the positive and negative symptoms of schizophrenia?

Ans. Positive symptoms refers to soft symptoms or excessive functioning symptoms in this individual's prognosis is good but in negative symptoms there will be diminished functioning and hard symptoms and the prognosis is poor:

	Positive Symptoms	Negative Symptoms
(i)	Ambivalence—holding two contradictory belief or feeling about same person/objective/event	Alogia—tendency to speak very little (Poverty of contents)
(ii)	Associative looseness poorly related thought and ideas	Anhedonia—feeling no joy or pleasure from life
(iii)	Delusion—false and fixed belief that have no basic in reality	Apathy—lack of social interaction
(iv)	Hallucination false sensory perception	Blunted affect—restricted range of emotional feeling tone or mood
(v)	Echolalia—automatic repetition of vocalizations made by another person	Avolitions—absence of will ambition or drive
(vi)	Echoproxia imitation of movement and gesture of another person	Catatonia—a period of agitation or excitement Flat affect—absence of facial expression

Q.8. What are the types of Schizophrenia?

Ans. There are following types of schizophrenia:

- Simple Schizophrenia
- Hebephrenic Schizophrenia (Disorganized schizophrenia)
- Catatonic Schizophrenia
- Paranoid Schizophrenia
- Undifferentiated Schizophrenia
- Residual Schizophrenia

- Acute Schizophrenic episode
- Schizo affective type
- Childhood type
- Post schizophrenic depression.

Q.9. Fill up the following:

1. Peak age of developing schizophrenia is ___________.
2. High incidence of schizophrenia is seen ___________ class people.
3. Deficiency of Vit ___________ and Vit ___________ is caused schizophrenia.
4. Silly behavior is seen is ___________ schizophrenic person.
5. Delusion of persecution; grandeur and idea of reference is found in ___________ schizophrenia.
6. Antipsychotic drugs are introduced in ___________.
7. ___________ Individual psychotherapy is most useful in schizophrenia.

Key

1. 25–30 year
2. Low socioeconomic
3. Vit B1, B6, B12
4. Hebephrenic
5. Paranoid
6. 1952
7. Reality oriented.

Q.10. What is difference between catatonic stupor and catatonic excitement?

Ans. Catatonic patient present catatonic stupor and catatonic excitement phase. Stupor phase follows depression apathy and patients become uncommunicative, characterized by failing interest, preoccupation in his own thought, emotional poverty. Patient become mute and mask like face. Patient can lie sit or stand in some position for days and weeks if not disturbed. Negativisim also present does not show any signs of painful stimuli.

In catatonic excitement phase patient behave in a wild and quite unpredictable manner patient shows aggressive motor activity. He/she may become agitated and can attack anyone near to him break and destroy articles flow of speech is usually ranges from flight of ideas, hallucination, etc.

Q.11. What intervention you will do for patient with delusion?

Ans. Following specific nursing intervention is useful to reduce client's delusion:

i. Do not argue with client, avoid comments
ii. Establish and maintain reality for the client
iii. Use distracting technique such as card playing
iv. Teach positive thinking.

Q.12. What are the nursing intervention can be carried out to reduce hallucination?

Ans. Following nursing intervention are useful to reduce hallucination:

1. Maintain good communication with client and maintain reality by frequent contact

2. Elicit description of hallucination to protect client and other
3. Diminish stimuli, such as noise, light and crowds around the patient
4. Engage client into diversional activity such as listening for music/card playing/ occupational activities, etc.
5. Reassure the client
6. Provide safety measures
7. Never alone the client-unlocked bathroom, no glass and bottles, ropes, medicine, nails in patient area.

Q.13. What are the treatment modalities for schizophrenia?

Ans. Treatment based on type of schizophrenia and severity of client is symptoms treatment includes following:

1. Psychopharmacology: A combination of antipsychotic, antidepressant, vitamin supplement, etc. is provided to reduce severity of symptoms.
2. Physical Therapy: ECT (Electro convulsive therapy).
3. Psychotherapy: Individual psycho—Reality oriented therapy.
4. Psychosocial therapy.

Q.14. How does social skill training is helpful in treatment of schizophrenia?

Ans. Social skill training has become one of most widely used psychosocial intervention in the treatment of schizophrenia.

Psychosocial skill training means a type of treatment based or principal of social learning theories to train and to retrain motor and interpersonal skill and competencies of client in these smaller set of behavior action and task are introduced and training retraining given to client.

The activity include—Daily living skill training such as bathing, brushing, dressing, grooming, purchasing, counting, banking marketing, traveling, etc. relaxation techniques yoga exercise, occupationally activities making paper bag craft candle making tailoring, etc.

Q.15. Fill up on antipsychotic drugs.

1. Antipsychotic drugs are introduced in .... (1952)
2. Antipsychotic drugs are also called .... (neuroleptics or major tranquilizer)
3. The most common antipsychotic drugs prescribed to patients are .... (chlorpromazine and butyrophenones halo peridol)
4. Antipsychotic drugs blocks .... (D2 receptor and histomine receptor blocks)
5. The common side effect of Antipsychotic drugs are .... (EPS extra pyramidal symptoms)
6. To prevent weight gain patient must not to take .... (caloric reached in beverage and candy)
7. To prevent photosensitivity patients must use .... (Sunscreen lotion protective clothing and goggles)
8. To avoid constipation patients is advise to increase .... (intake of water, roughages and exercise)
9. Convention non convention antipsychotic are .... (typical and atypical)
10. Endocrinal changes due to antipsychotic drug are .... (amenorrhea, weight gain and impotence)

Q.16. Which antipsychotic is best for patient?

Ans. Newer generation antipsychotic (i.e. Atypical antipsychotic) is best for Psychotic patient as these drugs have greater action and rare side effect like extrapyramidal syndrome.

Q.17. What is Dyskinesia?

Ans. Dyskinesia is a slow involuntary muscle contraction of jaw, neck, tongue, shoulder and trunk muscle. The patient maybe unable to open or close his mouth, difficulty in changing position. This can be treated by anticholinergic drugs.

Q.18. What is Akathisia?

Ans. Akathisia is a very common neuroleptic induced movement disorder, symptoms include inability to remain still, and complain of leg swinging, fast tapping, hand wringing with restless legs.

Q.19. What is Tardive Dyskinesia?

Ans. Tardive dyskinesia includes involuntary movements that may affect the mouth, lips tongue, arms, legs or trunk. It may occur due to long time administration of Antipsychotic drugs.

Q.20. What is neuroleptic malignant syndrome?

Ans. The Neuroleptic Malignant syndrome associated with antipsychotic medication, is characterized by fever (up to 107° f) severe, lead pipe rigidity, tachycardia labile blood pressure, diaphoresis. (This symptoms develop because of high dose of high potency antipsychotics) dehydration, malnourishment, etc.

Treatment consist of

- Stopping Antipsychotic
- Antipyretic therapy (Ice bath, cold water enema)
- Hydration with vitamin (IV therapy)
- Dantrolene 1 mg/kg (4–5 times/day)
- Bromocriptine (2.5 – 5 mg) oral three times a day.

Q.21. Enlist Endocrinal changes of antipsychotic drugs?

Ans. Endocrinal effects of Antipsychotic drugs are:

- Decreased erection
- Delayed ejaculation in males
- Menstrual irregularities in female
- Galactorrhea
- Weight gain
- Increased appetite, etc.

Q.22. Enlist role of nurse in antipsychotic medication.

Ans. Nursing responsibility of antipsychotic drugs administration are:

1. Provide treatment sips of water and oral hygiene to avoid mouth dryness
2. Do not administer drugs in empty stomach
3. Encourage use of high fibre diet to avoid constipation
4. Weigh the client every day
5. Advise client not to drive vehicle.

CHAPTER

28

Disorder of Mood and Affect

Q.1. Give one word answer:

1. Bipolar disorder is formerly known as
2. Which neurochemical deficiency causes depression
3. Which electrolyte responsible to cause depression
4. Increase level of serotonin and norepinephrine causes
5. Post stroke depression occur due to
6. Post stroke manic symptoms appear due to
7. Long terms use of which medicine cause bipolar disorder (depression and mania)
8. Which hormone is elevated is serum level of depressed client
9. Which vitamin deficiency causes depression
10. Which gender is mostly affected by bipolar disorder.

Key

1. Manic depressive illness
2. Norepinephrine and serotonin
3. Calcium and sodiumbicarbonate and potassium
4. Mania
5. Damage of left frontal lobe
6. Damage of right frontal temporal lobe
7. Steroids
8. Cortisol
9. Vitamin B1, B2, B12, and folic acid, vitamin C
10. Male.

Q.2. What are the Triad symptoms of depression and mania?

Ans. The Triad symptoms are:

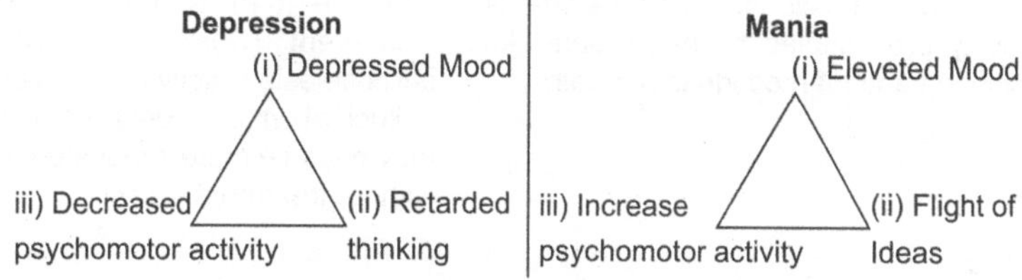

Q.3. What are the changes seen in Dietary habit and sleep pattern of depressive and manic patient?

Ans. In depressive patient does not shown self-interest towards intake of food, loss of appetite is seen and also weight loss can occur because of poor intake of diet. In mania because of increased motor activity and flight of ideas patient not able to sit in a place, not taking food in specific manner but eat in binge form and greedy type in sleep pattern depressive patient feel difficulty falling asleep usually at late night and late awaking is seen insomnia present in manic patient early falling asleep early awaking usually at midnight or early morning with full of energy and fresh mood.

Q.4. What are the other comparative features of mania and depression?

Ans. Comparative features

Depression	Mania
• Speech—Slow retarded content of speech some time become mute	Pressure of speech informal manner and high tone of speech
• Hygiene not interest to maintain self-care, bathing and dressing	Interested very much in maintaining personal hygiene and dressing grooming, colorful, bright dresses are select by patient and wear it in decorative manner
• Sex—Not interested in sexual activity	Hypersexual activity seen and homosexual is common in manic patient
• Activity—No social activity no talking to other people	Activity—Hyperactivity is seen talking to everyone
• IPR—Poor IPR with other	IPR – Interested to make IPR but not maintained
• Eye contact—No eye contact while talking other	Eye contact- Maintained eye contact
• Confidence—Low confidence low self-esteem feeling of guilt	Over confidence seen, spree bying Rackless driving, etc. seen
• Wants to be alone and feeling suicide thought	Wants to be in group violent and abusing
• Delusion—Nihilistic delusion or delusion of guilt is seen	Delusion of grandiosity seen

Q.5. What is the difference between depressive stupor and delirious mania?

Ans.

Depressive stupor	Delirious mania
It is most intensive form of depression patient presents with acute dementia, mute, and sensorium is clouded and he/she is intensively preoccupied he has dream like hallucination and marked ideas of death.	It is rare but fatal and dangerous form of mania. The patient is out of control. It is intensive form of mania in which speech incoherent (word salad) constantly and purposelesley activity is seen. Increased hallucination and delusion present patient may become more exhausted even may died without treatment.

Q.6. What is postpartum blue?

Ans. It is also called "Maternity blue" it is normal experience after delivery of a baby characterized by labile mood and affect, crying spell, sadness insomnia and anxiety. Symptoms begin approximately one day after delivery, usually peak in 3 to 7 days and disappear rapidly with no medical treatment.

Q.7. What is postpartum depression and postpartum psychosis?

Ans. Postpartum depressions occur within 4 weeks of postpartum, which meets all criteria of major depression. It is an emergency condition.

Postpartum psychosis is psychotic episode developing within 3 weeks of delivery beginning with fatigue, sadness, emotional liability, poor memory, confusion progressive to delusion hallucination, poor insight and judgment need medical treatment immediately.

Q.8. What is premenstrual dysphonic disorder?

Ans. Premenstrual dysphonic disorder is group of depressive symptoms occur before menses and subsided shortly after onset of menstruation. The features are as follows:

- Depressed mood, feeling hopelessness
- Anxiety, tension feeling of being "Keyed up"
- Increased sensitivity, suddenly sad labile mood
- Increased anger or irritability
- Decreased interest in usual activity work, school, friends or hobbies
- Lethargy, fatigability
- Insomnia or Hypersomnia
- Physical symptoms like breast tenderness or swelling headache, muscle pain, weight gain
- In above of the symptom at least 3 to 4 meet the criteria for diagnosis.

Q.9. Give meaning of following:

- Bipolar I disorder
- Bipolar II disorder
- Singing Mania
- Dancing Mania.
  - **Bipolar I disorder:** One or more mania or mixed episodes accompanied by major depressive episode
  - **Bipolar II disorder:** One or more major depressive episode accompanied by at least one hypomanic episode
  - **Singing mania:** Symptom of mania accompanied by rhyming and singing of patient
  - **Dancing mania:** Term used when client shows excessive happiness with increased motor activity followed by particular style of dance.

Q.10. Which antidepressant drugs are mostly prescribed by the psychiatrist and why?

Ans. The tricyclic antidepressant drugs (imipramine/amitriptyline, etc.) have been most widely prescribed than MAOIS drugs because MAOIS drug can cause Hypertensive crisis and has greater side effect than TCS produce sedative effect but it is mostly effective in treating depression.

Q.11. What are the action and nursing responsibility of antidepressant drugs?

Ans. Antidepressant drugs are classified as trycyclics, tetracyclics and MAO inhibitors, serotonin reuptake inhibitors, etc. Action of tricyclic antidepressant and MAO inhibitors increases neurotransmitters between nerve endings i.e. norepinephrine and serotonin in servotinin reuptake inhibitors block the action of mononine oxidize in breaking down excess of NE and 5HT at presynaptic neuron. Nursing responsibility of these drug include

- Do not administer at empty stomach and administer the drug at bedtime
- Discuss with patient that drug will be effective after 7–10 days of administration do not skip or change the dose by self
- Give plenty of oral fluid to prevent dryness of mouth
- Accurate recording of vital sign, i.e. BP and pulse to check orthostatic hypotension
- Record and maintain intake and output chart.

Q.12. Fill ups:

1. The drug of choice for acute mania and for maintainance therapy is _________.
2. Therapeutic level of lithium carbonate _________.
3. Toxic level of serum lithium is _________.
4. Pre-lithium work-up include _________ _________.
5. Other drug of treatment in mania includes _________.

Keys

1. Lithium Carbonate
2. 0.6 to 1.2 meq/L
3. 1.2 meq/L
4. ECG, LFT and RFT
5. Anticonvulsant and calcium channel blocker.

Q.13. What is lithium toxicity? What Nursing intervention will you do if patient develop toxicity?

Ans. Lithium toxicity is the most common side effect develop to sensitive patient after few days of lithium intake, it is increase level of lithium in blood produces various symptoms given in following table according to symptoms nurse should assess and intervention immediately.

Serum lithium level	Toxic symptoms	Nursing action
1 meq/L	Nausea, diarrhea, hand tremors malaise	• Stop next dose • Assess serum lithium • Inform to psychiatrist • Follow LFT, RFT • Start I/V fluid • Maintain I/o chart
1 to 2 meq/L	Drowsiness, vomiting, abdominal pain, lethargy dizziness, confusional ataxia	• Stop drug immediately • Assess serum lithium, LFT, RFT, ECG • Keep patient Nil orally

Contd...

Contd...

		• Start I/V fluid • Antiemetic, should administer maintain I/o chart strictly • Maintain fluid electrolyte imbalance • Keep safety and keen observation of patient
2 to 2.5 meq/L	Anorexia persistent nausea and vomiting blurred vision, seizure, acute circulatory failure oliguria, coma convulsion	• Above all action includes intensive care and patient must be posted for dialysis
Above 2.5	Generalize convulsion coma, oliguria and death	• General emergency care of patient includes resuscitation care

Q.14. Fill ups:

1. ____________ is a biological marker to distinguish individual with depression and post-traumatic stress disorder
2. _________ and _________ are self-report measures used to assess the presence of depression and severity of depression
3. ___________ is a useful in treatment of SAD seasonal affective disorder
4. Initial treatment for severely depress patient is __________.

Keys

i. Dexamethasone suppression test
ii. Beck depression inventory and Zung rating scale
iii. Light therapy
iv. ECT

CHAPTER 29

Anxiety Disorder

Q.1. What is anxiety? What are types of anxiety?

Ans. Anxiety is normal human emotion is experienced in varying degrees as a state of emotion or physical uneasiness level of anxiety is:

The triad symptoms are

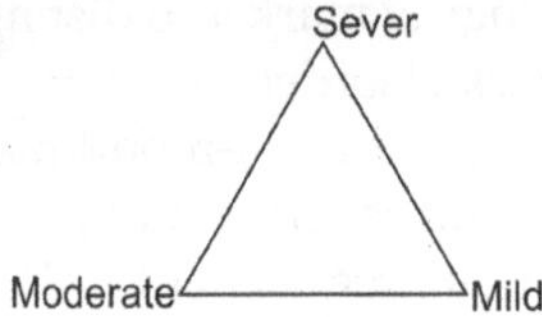

Q.2. What are the features of anxiety?

Ans. Features of anxiety at different level are

Physiological level:

- Increase Heart Rate
- Elevated BP
- Palpitation
- Pain and tightness in chest
- Breathing difficulty
- Sweating, sleep disturbance

Cognitive (Intellectual) level:

- Forgetfulness
- Poor judgment
- Decreased concentration
- Decreased productivity

Emotion and Affective:

- Irritability
- Feeling of sadness and depression
- Helplessness and hopelessness.

Q.3. Define Phobia.

Ans. "Phobia" is persistent avoidance behavior. Secondary to irrational fear of a specific object activity or situation.

Q.4. What is Panic disorder?

Ans. It is sever form of anxiety characterized by spontaneous unexpected occurrence of panic attacks (usually less than one hour) period of anxiety or fear accompanied by somatic symptoms like palpitation and tachypnea (clinical features are listed above).

Q.5. Enlist the type of phobia?

Ans. Types of phobia are as follows:

Agoraphobia	Specific Phobia	Social Phobia
Fear to crowded stores, closed in space (tunnels, rides and elevators etc.)	Fear to specific object like (height, water, animal, darkness etc.)	Fear to expose in to public or social situation (stage performance)

Q.6. What is obsessive-compulsive disorder?

Ans. Obsessions are persistent ideas, thoughts impulses or images that are recurrent and intrusive cause anxiety, compulsion are behavior or mental acts designed to prevent or reduce anxiety or distress compulsive rituals are counting checking, cleaning, washing, etc.

Q.7. What is Generalized Anxiety Disorder (GAD)?

Ans. Generalized Anxiety Disorder is chronic lifelong mild to moderate form of anxiety existing one to two year with symptoms of nervousness, trembling, muscular tension, sweating, light headness, etc.

Q.8. What is Post-traumatic Stress Disorder PTSD?

Ans. Post-traumatic Stress Disorder is a delayed and or protracted response to stressful events or situation of an exceptionally threatening or catastrophic nature.

Q.9. What is Dissociative (Conversion) Disorders?

Ans. Dissociative (conversion) disorder was previously known as hysteria referred to physical or mental symptoms not of organic origin created and maintained for unconscious psychological motives and associated with somatoform disorders (do not associated with physical basic).

- It is defined as partial completed loss normal integration between memories of post, awareness of identity and immediate sensation and control of bodily movements main types are:
  - Dissociative amnesia
  - Dissociative stupor
  - Dissociative fugue.

Q.10. What are the biological causes of panic disorder?

Ans. Panic disorder is caused by certain biological factors such as:

1. High level of lactate in blood induces hyperventilation
2. High amount of carbon dioxide in blood also cause hyperventilation-alarming suffocation
3. Increased level of norepinephrine also cause panic attack leads symptoms of tachycardia and palpitation
4. Abnormally in serotonin level
5. GABA: excessive release of GABA cause panic anxiety
6. Limbic system dysfunction cause anxiety disorder.

Q.11. What is the treatment of anxiety disorder?

Ans. Client suffering with Anxiety disorder receive combination of treatment:

a. Antianxiety drugs (Benzodiaepines): Alprazolam (2 to 6 mg daily in divided dose) diazepam is longer acting drug given in 1 to 4 mg twice daily in devided dose

b. Antidepressant drugs: SSRIS and TCAS are effective in reducing the frequency and severity of panic attacks

c. Cognitive behaviour: Therapy used to decrease negative thought and bringing up positive thoughts
d. Paradoxical intention: In this therapy therapist instruct the client to hyperventilate or actually bring on a panic attack by ceasing struggle to prevent anxiety. The individual gains a sense of control over and tolerance for the discomfort
e. Exposure therapy: Flooding the most intense of the intervention either in imagery or in the environment of anxiety provoking stimuli without relaxation or pause until anxiety subsides
f. Exposure and response prevention: It is the treatment of OCD in this client is exposure to the stimulus causing obsession (such as contamination of hand) and ask to do activity (Compulsion) but time has to limit by the therapist.

Q.12. Enlist Nursing Intervention for the client with anxiety disorder?

Ans. Nursing intervention for patient with anxiety disorder are:
- Interact with the client in a calmer manner
- Use soft voice and reassuring approach reduce stimuli
- Listen to the client's concerns
- Teach relaxation technique such as deep breathing muscle relaxation
- Administer antianxiety drugs
- Teach to avoid caffeine, nicotine and stimulant substance like alcohol.

Q.13. What are the nursing activities for phobic patient?

Ans. Nursing Activities are:
- Understand that phobic responses are irrational and will not be changed by logical explanation
- Listen and acknowledge the client's fear and emotion in a supportive and non-judgmental manner
- Use technique of Role-play to control anxiety
- Discuss alternative ways to control phobic response.

Q.14. Enlist nursing intervention for the patient with post-trauma response:

Ans. Post-trauma response is evidenced by flashback, nightmares, increased anxiety symptoms related to traumatic events such as rape, car accident or war, etc. The nurse has to perform important and sensitive activities as follows:
- Encourage venting feeling of fear, anger and powerlessness in a supportive reassuring environment.
- Provide trusting environment without showing judgment or shock during this process.
- Teach relaxation technique as a way to relieve anxiety and tension.
- Encourage to development of new skill and alternatives to more quickly adoption.
- Assist and support the client with legal and medical issues as appropriate.

Q.15. What are the features of dissociative amnesia?

Ans. The main feature of dissociative amnesia is loss of memory, usually of important recent event:
- Forgetfulness or fatigue
- Distress
- Local wondering.

Q.16. Enlist features of dissociative fugue.

Ans. All feature of dissociative amnesia included purposeless journey away from home or place of work.

Q.17. What are the symptoms of dissociative motor disorder?

Ans. Symptoms include loss of ability to move the whole or a part of a limb:

- Partial paralysis
- Trembling or shaking of one or more extremities or the whole body.

Q.18. Define Somatoform disorder.

Ans. Somatoform disorder is defined as the use of physical symptoms to express emotional problems and psychosocial stress.

Q.19. What is hypochondriasis?

Ans. Hypochondriasis is characterized by a preoccupation with fear of having or developing a serious physical illness. The disorder is often chronic, symptoms present for months or years.

Q.20. Who are the high-risk group for PTSD?

Ans. High-risk group for PTSD are:

- Children
- Disabled people
- Elderly

Women, young, single, widowed orphaned, disabled orphaned, childhood abuse, etc.

Q.21. Give meaning of following terms related to PTSD?

a. Flash back: Acting or feeling as if the event were actually happening intrusive re-experiencing of the traumatic event.

b. Hyper vigilance: Close attention to and anticipation of approaching danger.

c. Avoidance: Efforts to avoid thoughts, feeling or conversation associated with trauma.

d. Numbness: A condition of being detached indifferent and devoid of feeling particularly for traumatic event.

Fill ups

a. __________ is useful to relieve symptoms of PTSD.

b. __________ or __________ may reduce intrusive symptoms of PTSD.

c. __________ reduce the symptoms of anxiety and hyper arousal.

d. In acute stress condition increased amount of __________ are secreted.

e. Extreme stress has deleterious effect on __________ and __________.

Keys

a. Fluoxetine

b. Propranolol or Clonidine

c. Bezodiazepines

d. Cortisol

e. Hippocampus and Limbic systems

CHAPTER

30

Substance Abuse and Alcoholism

Q.1. Give meaning of following terminology:

Ans. **a. Psychotropic:** The word referes to "exerting an effect on the mind"

b. Psychotropic substance: Psychoactive/psychotropic substance are drugs or chemical that when taken alter one or several of the following symptoms, perception, awareness, consciousness, thinking, judgment, decision-making, insight, mood and behavior

c. Drug abuse: A pathological use of drug or alcohol with impairment in social, personal, occupational functioning

d. Drug dependence: A state of physical or psychological compulsion to take drug on continuous bases

e. Physical dependence: Without drugs person may experience symptoms of mild to moderate discomfort which relieved by taking drugs

f. Psychological dependence: When drugs are being used for central to thought, emotion, activities, individual have craving for it

g. Withdrawal: It is group of symptom following cessation (stopping) or reduction in the intake of a substance such as alcohol on opoid, amphetamine, etc. symptoms of anxiety, restlessness, insomnia impaired attention and irritability.

Match the following: Psychotropic drugs and their effect:

	A		B
1	Alcohol	A	Stimulation alertness
2	Diazepam	B	Blackouts
3	Cocanine	C	Drowsiness sedation
4	Nicotine	D	Euphoria wake fullness
5	Morphine	E	Pinpoint pupils analgesia
6	Cannabis	F	Panic attack paranoia
7	Caffeine	G	Increased blood pressure enhanced performance
8	LSD	H	Altered perception (bad trip)

Keys

1	B	2	C
3	F	4	G
5	E	6	D
7	A	8	H

Q.2. Enlist physiological symptoms of drug dependence.

Ans. Malnutrition

- Gastritis's
- Hepatomegaly
- Hypertension
- Cardiomegaly
- COPD
- Tremors, peripheral neuropathy nystagmus ataxia ophthalmologic myopathy.

Q.3. What are mental changes occur due to drugs abuse?

Ans. Following mental changes occur:

- Hallucination, delusion, illusion
- Delirium
- Insomnia
- Manic symptoms, suspicious of wife's fidelity.

Q.4. What are the general management of drug overdose?

Ans. Take vital signs:

- Assess and maintain adequate airway and respiration
- Maintain circulation
- Obtain complete history of use of alcohol hypnotic, sedative, opiates, drug
- Obtain physical examination level of consciousness, history of trauma, alcohol breath
- Obtain general test CBC, electrolyte, LFT, RFT, urine routine, etc.
- Monitor intake and output chart
- Administer IV fluid to maintain fluid electrolytes balance
- Initiate gastric levage
- Watch for sign of intoxication
- Arrange intensive care.

Q.5. What are the signs of Benzodiazepine overdose and its treatment?

Ans. Signs of Benzodiazepine overdose include:

- Mild to moderate CNS depression.
- Drowsiness
- Sedation

Treatment: Flumazeniel 0.3 mg to 0.5 mg every 30 sec. to 1 minute up to 5 mg 1 mg bolus dose 3 mg/hr.

Q.6. What are the sign of opiate intoxication? What is the treatment of it?

Ans. Sign of stupor, respiratory depression urinary retention decreased peristalsis

Treatment: Naloxone is an opiate antagonist 0.4 mg IV to 2 mg IV

- Naloxone 2 mg in 500 ml in 5% dextrose saline infusion over 15–20 minutes

Q.7. Write signs of alcohol intoxication. What is the treatment?

Ans. Severe alcohol intoxication results in loss of inhibition, stupor coma

- CNS depression
- Hypoglycemia
- Thiamine deficiency
- Neuropathy

T/t: Inj. thiamine 100 mg IV with 50% dextrose

All general medical treatment

Q.8. Enlist symptoms of alcohol withdrawal.

Ans. Withdrawal symptoms occur within 48 hrs of alcohol cessation symptoms are:

- Insomnia, vivid dreaming
- Sweating tachycardia
- Anxiety tremors
- Nausea vomiting
- Alcoholic seizures (5 to 15% of people)
- Delirium psychosis hallucination, etc.

Treatment: Admit the client into hospital

- Require carefully observation
- Decrease stimulation
- Administer IV fluid maintain hydration and electrolyte balance
- Carry out general and specific physical examination
- Add vitamin, thiamine 100 mg IM then orally daily folic acid 1 mg orally 7–10 days.
- Administer Benzodiazepine (Librium/Diazepine) chlordia-zepoxide 10 mg (Librium) is equivalent to diazepam 5 mg
- Administer Antipsychotic Haloperidol 5–20 mg orally to reduce hallucination
- Psychotherapy: Motivational interview to be initiate to control the client habbit.

Q.9. How deaddiction is done from alcohol?

Ans. Disulfiram (antabuse therapy) therapy is used to make client abstinence from alcohol.

Actions: Disulfiran is an aldehyde dehydrogeniz inhibitor that interferes with alcohol metabolism and produce high acetaldehyde level it produce reaction called DER disulfiran ethanol reaction symptom include throbbing headache, nausea vomiting abdominal cramps facial flushing tachycardia, etc.

Nursing Responsibility: Obtain informed consent before starting the therapy

- Ensure to stop ingestion of alcohol before 12 hrs of therapy
- Restrict alcohol containing food sauce, remover, jelly, cough syrup, etc.
- Assess all physiological test CBC, LFT, RFT, ECG, etc.
- Strict intake output charting
- Patients should provide identification card.

Q.10. Give one word answers of following:

1. Period of amnesia after alcohol intake is called __________.
2. Sever memory loss due to thiamine deficiency in alcohol client is term as __________.
3. Hallucination due to alcohol effect is __________.
4. Treatment of korsakoff psychosis is __________.
5. 80–100 mg/100 ml of alcohol in blood produce __________.
6. Disullfiram is an __________.
7. An easily approachable screening questionnaire for alcoholic client is __________.

Keys

1. Blackout
2. Korsakoff psychosis
3. Alcoholic psychosis
4. Vitamin thiamine
5. Intoxication
6. Acetaldehyde dehydrogenase enzyme inhibitor
7. CAGE questionnaire.

CHAPTER 31

Eating and Personality Disorder

Q.1. Define Personality disorder.

Ans. According to DSM IV when personality traits are inflexible and maladaptive cause either significant functional impairment or subjective distress.

Q.2. Enlist classification of personality disorder.

Ans. ICD-10 (f60-f69) classify personality disorder as follows:

i. Paranoid PD
ii. Schizoid PD
iii. Dissocial PD (Antisocial)
iv. Emotionally unstable PD
v. Impulsive type Borderline type
vi. Histrionic PD
vii. Anankastic PD (Obsessive-compulsive)
viii. Anxious Avoidant
ix. Dependent
x. Other specific PD (Narcissistic PD)

DSM IV (R) classification

i. **Cluster–A** (odd and Eccentric Personality disorder (PDS) thought to be an Schizophrenic)
   a. Paranoid personality disorders.
   b. Schizoid personality disorders.
   c. Schizotypal personality disorder.
ii. **Cluster – B** (Dramatic, emotional and erratic)
   a. Antisocial personality disorder
   b. Historionic personality disorders
   c. Narcisstic personality disorders
   d. Borderline personality disorders
iii. **Cluster – C** (Anxious and fearful)
   a. Avoidant personality disorders
   b. Dependent personality disorders
   c. Obsessive compulsive personality disorders.

Q.3. Match the characteristic of following personality disorder:

A	B
1. Individual with suspicious and mistrustful	a. Antisocial personality
2. Emotional coldness shy detachment from reality	b. Paranoid personality
3. Very low tolerance to frustration	c. Schizoid personality
4. Attention seeking behavior, over involvement dramatic	d. Obsessive compulsive disorder
5. Excessive doubt and caution preoccupation with rules, list, order	e. Histrionic personality
6. Individual exhibit symptoms of extreme anxiety and fear in social and intimate relationship	f. Dependent personality
7. Unable to make independent decision	g. Anxious Avoidant Personality

Key:

1 – b, 2 – c, 3 – a, 4 – e, 5 – d, 6 – g, 7 – f

Q.4. Fill ups:

i. __________ discovered personality disorder.
ii. __________ Psychotherapy is useful for paranoid personality disorder.
iii. __________ and __________ is used to treat Antisocial personality disorder.
iv. In anxious (avoidant) personality disorder __________ is choice of psychotherapy.
v. __________ therapy is treatment of choice in dependent personality disorder.
vi. __________ is used to treat borderline personality disorder.

Ans. (i) James Pritchard, (ii) Supportive psychotherapy, (iii) Self-help group and therapeutic community, (iv) Assertiveness, (v) Dynamic, (vi) CBT cognitive – behavior therapy.

Q.5. What is Paraphilias?

Ans. It is disorder of sexual preference characterized by recurrent intense urges, fantasies or behavious that involve unusual object, activities, or situation and causes or impairment is social occupational or other important areas of functioning.

Give meaning of following:

i. **Transexualism:** A desire to live and be accepted as a member of the opposite sex, usually accompanied by a sense of discomfort with or inappropriateness of ones' anatomic sex and a wish to have hormonal treatment and surgery to make one's body as congruent as possible with the preferred sex
ii. **Transvestism:** Wearing of clothes of opposite sex for part of the individual's existence in order to enjoy the temporary experience of membership of the opposite sex but without desire for a permanent sex change
iii. **Fetishism:** Reliance on some non-living object as stimulus for sexual arousal and sexual gratification many fetishes are extension of human body. Such as articles of clothing or footwear mainly seen in males
iv. **Fetishistic transvestism:** The wearing of clothes of the opposite sex principally to obtain sexual excitement
v. **Exhibitionism:** A recurrent or persistent tendency to expose to genitals to strangers (usually of opposite sex)

vi. **Voyeurism:** A recurrent or persistent tendency to look at people engaging in sexual or intimate behavior such as undressing

vii. **Pedophilia:** A sexual preference for children usually of prepubertal or early pubertal age

viii. **Dyspareunia:** Dyspareunia is characterized by recurrent or persistent genital pain associated with sexual intercourse in either a male or a female which causes marked distress.

Q.6. What is anorexia nervosa?

Ans. Anorexia nervosa is a psychiatric disorder characterized by a voluntary refusal to eat.

Q.7. What is the Neuropathological cause of anorexia Nervosa?

Ans. Decreased activity of central nervous system and low level of neurotransmitter (NE) and low level of dopamine also play role in anorexia nervosa.

Q.8. Short Answer Questions:

I. The cardinal feature of anorexia nervosa is:

Ans. Body weight less than 85% of normally expected for age and height.

II. Preoccupation associated with anorexia nervosa is:

Ans. Body weight and body shape.

III. Which clinical feature is helpful to diagnosing anorexia nervosa in girl client:

Ans. History of amenorrhea and nutritional deprivation.

IV. In man endocrinal signs of anorexia nervosa involved is:

Ans. Loss of sexual interest and impotency.

V. Preoccupied thought with eating and irresistible craving for food seen in?

Ans. Bulimia nervosa.

VI. Patient with bulimia nervosa attempts to counteract the overfeeding by which method.

Ans. Self-induced vomiting or purgative abuse or alternating period of starvation.

VII. Hypersecretion of which hormone causing decrease metabolism in-patient with anorexia nervosa.

Ans. Excessive production of cortisol.

VIII. What is reason of having impaired thermal regulation in anorexia nervosa?

Ans. Hypothyroidism (Decreased level of T3 Hormone Tri-iodothyronin).

IX. Which gland is hyperstimulated in bulimia nervosa?

Ans. Parotid and salivary gland.

Q.9. Enlist nursing intervention for the client with eating disorder.

Ans. The main goal of a nurse is to achieve normal nutritional status for client so that she should plan and initiate following action:

- Make therapeutic contract with the client regarding time, frequency and procedure for weighing the patient
- Explain the client about time of meal and amount of time allotted to each meal
- Instruct the amount of water that client must be drink each day
- Make schedules for meal timing
- Select their own menu
- Cooking food for them with supervision
- Set a realistic goal of gaining weight 1 pound per week
- Teach the effect of proper nutrition
- Teach proper eating habits.

CHAPTER 32

Mental Retardation

Q.1. Define mental retardation.

Ans. Mental retardation is a condition of incomplete development of intellectual functioning it is not a disease but condition in which the intellectual ability have never been developed sufficiently.

It is defined as:

"Significantly deficit or impairment in adaptive functioning, i.e. person's ability to meet the responsibilities of social, personal, interpersonal and occupational areas of life according to his age and sociocultural and educational background."

Q.2. What is the formula to obtain IQ of a person?

Ans. The degree or level of mental retardation is obtained by the ratio of

$$IQ = \frac{\text{Mental age} \times 100}{\text{Chronological age}} \quad \text{For example} \quad \frac{3}{10} \times 100$$

IQ = 30

Q.3. What are different levels of mental retardation?

Ans. According to ICD-X. Level of mental Retardation depends on severity of degree of mental function.

i. Mild – Mental Retardation (IQ–50–69) mental age of this group is 9–12 years
ii. Moderate mental Retardation (35–49) mental age 6–9 years
iii. Sever mental retardation (IQ 20–34) mental age 3–6 years
iv. Profound mental retardation (IQ less than 20) mental age less than 3 years.

Q.4. What are etiological factors of mental retardation?

Ans. Cause of mental retardation are as follows:

- Prenatal causes: Infection (Rubella, Syphilis, Cytomegalovirus).
- Physical damage – (Injury, hypoxia, radiation).
- Intoxication (lead, certain drugs).
- Antenatal poor nutrition toxemia of pregnancy.

Intranatal Causes:

- Birth asphyxia
- Prologed labor
- Obstructed labor
- Preterm baby
- Instrumental delivery

Postnatal Damage
- Injury (Accident, child abuse)
- Infection

Genetic Disorder

Down syndrome–Trisomy–21

Metabolic Disorder

Amino acid disorder (Phenyl ketonuria)

Brain Disease – Multiple selerosis, hydrocephaly

Sociocultural deprivation.

Q.5. What are the clinical feature of mental retardation?

Ans. The most characteristic signs are as follows:
- Four of these features are accepted as strong evidence for the syndrome
- Mouth: Small mouth and teeth furrowed tongue, high arched palate
- Eyes: Epicanthic folds
- Head: Flat occiput
- Hands: Short and broad, single transverse crease
- Joints: Hyperextensibility, hypoxia
- Others: Congenital heart disease, small dysplastic ear, impaired hearing, occular disturbance, etc.

Q.6. What are management and prevention taken to treat mental retardation?

Ans. No satisfactory treatment is available till today. No drugs are available to increase the level of intelligence. Symptomatic treatments are given to children are benefited to some extent only. Management can be directed at following level.

Primary Prevention	Secondary Prevention	Tertiary Prevention
(a) Health promotion	***Early diagnosis and treatment***	***Disability limitation***
• Good Antenatal care and encouraging hospital deliveries • General Awareness to public to help early detection of mentally retardation.	• Detection of high-risk pregnancy • Detection of nutritional and endocrinal disorder • Amniocentesis and MTP at medical ground • Tubectomy of severely Retarded girls.	• Treatment of physical and psychological problems (with drugs and behavior modification) • Education and training retraining to moderately retarded child • Physiotherapy to treat associated deficit • Special school teaching rehabilitation: Social skill training at day care centre special school, vocational training to make them-self sufficient like candle making, tailoring, etc. with supervision. • Provide support and security by family member

Contd...

ntd...

(b) Specific protection:	*General nursing care:*	
• Good potential, antenatal and postnatal care to the pregnant mother at risk • Genetic counseling to risk couples • Avoid late marriage and consanguine marriage • Avoid marriage of mentally retarded. • Rubella vaccination to adolescent girls • Avoid exposure to radiation, poision during pregnancy state. • Avoid trauma during natal period	• Maintain hygiene of child to avoid any infection • Well balanced diet to maintain normal physical growth • Well dressing • Teaching small activity to engage them • Mental assessment to detect any other mental abnormality	

Q.7. Short Answers Question:

1 Which group is called Trainable group?

Ans. Moderately mentally Retardated group (IQ 35 to 50).

2. Which group is educable group?

Ans. Mild degree (IQ 50 to 70) of mental retardation.

3. Which group is called dependent group?

Ans. Severe degree of mental retardation (IQ 20–35).

4. Which chromosomal abnormality found mostly in mentally retarded child?

Ans. Down's Syndrome (Trisomy 21)

5. Which invasive procedure is done in ANC women to rule out genetic abnormalities?

Ans. Amniocentesis and chorionic villi biopsy.

6. To measure IQ level which test is used generally:

Ans. Standford Binet IQ Test.

7. First teacher training for graduate teacher's for the education of physically of handicapped children started at

Ans. Mumbai in 1977

8. Name few centre providing residence and care for mentally retarded child:

Ans. ENRICH (Wilson Garden Bangalore)

- Spastic Society of Karnataka
- Ashakiran (Bangalore)
- Arpana Special School (Bangalore)
- Bethany Special School
- Sneh Sampada (Chhattisgarh, Bhilai)
- Prayash (School for deaf and dumb) Chhattisgarh Bhilai
- Sangath Society (GOA)
- Samadhan (New Delhi).

CHAPTER 33

Organic Brain Disorder

Q.1. What is the meaning of organic brain disorder?

Ans. The term "Organic" means that the syndrome can be attributed to cerebral or systemic disease.

Organic mental disorder is a psychological or behavioral abnormality associated with transient or permanent dysfunction of brain.

Q.2. What are the types of organic brain disorder?

Ans. According to ICD–X it has many classification but in general it is of few types:

i. Acute, e.g. Delirium
ii. Chronic, e.g. Dementia

Others are organic hallucinosis
Organic catatonic disorder
Organic delusional disorder
Organic manic disorder
Organic anxiety disorder
Organic personality disorder.

Q.3. Define dementia.

Ans. According ICD–X "Dementia is a syndrome due to disease of the brain usually of a chronic or progressive nature in which there is disturbance of multiple higher cortical function, including, memory, thinking, orientation comprehension calculation, learning capacity, language and judgment.

Q.4. What is the pathophysiology of dementia?

Ans. Pathophysiology varies on the basic cause of dementia in Alzheimer's there is decrease level of neuron's in hippocampus substantial temporoparietal and frontal cortex and decreased enzyme in choline acetyltransferase. In infarct vascular changes occur due to decrease blood supply and O_2 to cerebral tissue that leads to brain dysfunction.

Q.5. What are stages of dementia?

Ans. Dementia is progressive in nature it has mainly seven stages occur during Alzheimer Dementia:

Stage I	–	No decline in memory
Stage II	–	Early stage of forget fullness like forgetting name of people
Stage III	–	Early confusion decreased concentration at work place
Stage IV	–	Late confusion forget major events like date of birth date of wedding etc.
Stage V	–	Early dementia stage remain for 2–4 years decrease ability to independent ADL and Job performance
Stage VI	–	Middle dementia person may be unable to recall recent major events even forget name of spouse.
Stage VII	–	Late dementia progressive memory loss with disturbance in physiological function even he becomes bed ridden.

Q.6. What are the clinical features of dementia?

Ans. 3A features of dementia are

Aphasia – Deterioration of language

Apraxia – Impaired ability to execute motor function

Agnosia – Inability to recognize or name object

Other Symptoms are:

- Loss of memory
- Loss of ability to think and plan initiate and monitoring
- Cannot attend more than one stimulus at time
- Depression, confusion isolation and withdrawal.

Q.7. What are the nursing intervention to be provided for dementia client?

Ans. Nursing intervention to be provide at hospital, home care and rehabilitation

- **Improving personal hygiene:** Encourage and support self-care active bathing, dressing, etc.
- **Improving nutrition:** Patient feel difficulty in swallowing chewing encourage to chew first in one side of the mouth and then on the Other. Increase calorie intake by supplementary food
- Massaging facial and neck muscle before meals
- Improving bowel elimination: Avoid constipation increase fluid intake and fiber rich diet and regular exercise
- **Improve communication:** Use simple conversation (e.g. Yes/No.) encourage successful communication to patient
- Sentence should be short and literal
- **Improving mobility:** Encourage and assist daily exercise to increase muscle strength (Active, passive exercise)
- **Enhancing memory:** Use memory aids written reminders placed in strategic places such as locking the door or turning off the iron
- **Use object clues:** Telephonic reminder and memory tapes, etc. Use music therapy for sensory stimulation
- **Improve sleep:** Client with dementia may sleep periodically throughout the day and be awake all Night. Few nursing intervention are important to enhance sleep pattern
- Keep the patient active throughout the day
- Discourage them from taking naps at daytime

- Establish a bedtime routine
- Place the patient in safe, dim lighted bedroom encourage to listen light music or playing cards to induce sleep
- Provide warm bath or light snacks warm milk at bedtime
- Remove object which create hallucination.

Q.8. One Word Answer:

1. Name the therapy used for dementia patient to experiencing the world and deriving pleasure and sensory stimulating?

Ans. Remotivation therapy.

2. In which therapy nurse enters in the world of patient to understand him/her to reduce incidence of agitation and catastrophic reaction?

Ans. Validation therapy.

3. Which drug is prescribed to increase anticholinesterase agent to improve memory of dementia client?

Ans. Tab Tacrine.

4. Which Antipsychotic is best for treating signs of agitation and aggression associated with dementia?

Ans. Tab Haloperidol
Tab Risperidone
Tab Olanzapine.

5. Which drugs are used to reduce symptoms of insomnia?

Ans. Short acting benzodiazepines.

CHAPTER 34

Psychiatric Emergency

Q.1. What is psychiatric emergency?

Ans. Psychiatric emergency is a condition where in the patient has the disturbances of thought affect and psychomotor activity leading to treat to his existence or threat to the people in the environment.

Q.2 What are psychiatric emergency conditions?

Ans. The common psychiatric emergency are:
- Suicide
- Violence
- Stupor
- Panic
- Withdrawal symptoms of (drugs and alcohol)
- Drug intoxication and alcohol/intoxication
- Delirium
- Hysterical fits
- Hyperventilation
- Amnesia
- Severe depression
- Side effects of psychotropic drugs
- EPS
- Dystonia
- Akathisia
- Lithium toxicity
- Stressful situation.

Q.3. What are the preventive strategies for Suicide?

Ans. Suicide: Suicide is not a disease or disorder but it is behavior of intentional taking of one's life in a culturally non-endorsed manner.

Management tips for suicidal client.

Assess following:
- Every suicide ideation, gesture, impulse or attempt should be taken seriously
- The patient should asked to discuss freely his feelings
- Enquire feelings of depression and hopelessness

- Be aware of nonverbal communication
- Remove all sharp object, material from surrounding including drugs and poisons
- Never leave patient alone
- If there is medicolegal problem inform to police (Rape, Abuse)
- Take help of crisis hot lines services
- Counseling and support instilling hope
- Administer mild tranquilizer 5–10 mg diazepam or lorazepam 1–2 mg at night for calming anxiety and stress.

Q.4. How do you manage violent patient?

Ans. Violence is physical aggression by one person on another It is most commonly associated with psychotic disorder management tips for violent patient

i. Remove all sharp object from surrounding.
ii. Do not sit close to patient.
iii. Keeps the doors open.
iv. Do restraint physically if necessary.
v. Do not confront.
vi. Give medicine
   a. Chlorpromazine 50–150 mg. IM with or without promethazine. (25 to 50 mgs)
   b. Haloperidol 5 to 10 mg (IM/IV) with or without promethazine Rapid Neuroleptization with Haloperidol 20 mg IV and repeat every 20 mts to 1 hr. maximum of 120 mg/day till the violence or aggressive behavior is controlled
   c. Diazepam 10 to 40 mg IV slowly till patient's violent behavior is controlled
vii. Counseling and reassure the client.

CHAPTER 35

Psychotherapeutic Modalities

Q.1. What is ECT?

Ans. Electroconvulsive therapy is a type of somatic treatment in which electric current is applied to the brain through electrodes. Placed on the temporal region of the patient. The passage of an electrical stimulus of 70 to 150 volts to the brain for 0.1 to 0.5 second to produce a grandmal seizure.

Q.2. Who introduced ECT first time?

Ans. ECT was first introduced in 1934 but in April 1938 Bini and Cerletti in Rome administered successfully to a man of 39 years old.

Q.3. What is a mechanism of action of ECT?

Ans. The exact mechanism is unknown but it is thought to produce biochemical changes in the brain it increase level of norepinphrine and serotonin similar to the effects of antidepressant medications.

Q.4. What are the Indications of electroconvulsive therapy?

Ans. Following are indications for ECT:

Major severe depression	Severe catatonia	Sever psychosis
Sever depression with suicidal risk	With Stupor	Schizophrenia
With stupor	Poor intake of diet	Mania
Melancholia	Unsatisfactory response of drug	Suicide
Psychotic feature	Where drug is contra Indicated or have serious side effects.	Schizoaffective disorder
Unsatisfactory to drug therapy		Where drugs are contraindicated.
Serious side effect of anti-depressant drugs		Unsatisfactory to drug response

Q.5. In which condition ECT is contraindicated?

Ans. ECT is contraindicated in following condition:

1. Raised Intracranial pressure
2. History of cerebral infarct aneurysm
3. Myocardial infarction

4. Brain tumor
5. Cardiac disease
6. Respiratory disease (TB Asthma)
7. CVA
8. CCF
9. Retinal detechment

Q.6. What are the techniques of ECT?

Ans. The Techniques used for ECT administration of two types.

1. Direct ECT
2. Modified ECT

In Direct ECT: It is given in the absence of muscular relaxation and general anesthesia. This is now infrequently used because of convulsion patient and relatives both are feel shocked and afraid

Modified ECT: In Modified ECT drugs induced muscular relaxation and general anesthesia used.

Q.7. What are frequency and volt used in ECT?

Ans. The volts of electrical stimulus is from 70 to 150 volts, for 0.1 to 0.5 second to produce grandmal seizure.

Frequency of ECT depends upon client condition, severity of clinical feature, etiological factor and physical status of patient. Usually two or three per week is prescribed.

Q.8. What are the types of ECT?

Ans. There are two types of administration:

1. Bilateral
2. Unilateral

Bilateral ECT: This is the standard form of ECT most commonly used, which bilateral ECT electrodes are placed on each side one inch above the midpoint of an imaginary line connecting the outer canthus of the eye and targus of ear

Unilateral ECT electrodes are placed only on one side of head usually right side of head in a right handed individual

Unilateral is a safer, with fewer side-effects particularly those of memory impairment.

Q.9. What are the pre-ECT nursing responsibilities?

Ans. Following are pre-ECT nursing responsibilities:

- Assess all physical mental assessment prior ECT
- Informed consent must be taken prior to ECT
- Check and record all essential laboratory work
- Keep nil orally 6–8 hours before ECT
- Stop anticonvulsant and sedative (like carbomazepine, phenobarb, etc.) before night ECT
- Remove dentures, glasses, jewelry, contact lens, metal hair clips, pins from patient
- Dress the patient in loose garments
- Instruct client to empty bladder and bowel
- Monitor and record vital signs before during and after treatment
- Keep all emergency drugs and equipment ready for resuscitive purpose

Q.10. What are the Post-ECT functions of nurses?

Ans. Post ECT functions of nurses are as follows:
- Observe and record the respiration pulse and blood pressure of the patient
- Put railing and place the patient on a side lying position, wipe the secretion
- Transfer the patient to the recovery room only when client is respond verbal command
- Watch, record vitals every 15 to 30 minutes till patient recovers fully
- Allow patient to sleep for 30 minutes to 1 hour
- Reorient the client to ward toilet and nursing stations
- Watch for any physical complain or pain
- Encourage patient to take bath and change his/her cloth
- Allow to take clear tea with light breakfast.

Q.11. What are the articles required for ECT?

Ans. Nurse must be responsible to see all sufficient articles required for ECT procedure are as follows:
- ECT machine in working condition
- Jelly and electrodes
- BP Apparatus
- Intubations set
- Anesthesia trolley containing suction apparatus, mask, tongue depressor, resuscitation apparatus
- Mouth gag, gauze pieces, cotton swab, kidney tray
- O2 cylinder
- Injection sodium pentathol
- Succinylcholine
- Atropine sulfate
- Diazepam
- Anticholinergic drugs.

Q.12. What are the side effect of ECT?

Ans. ECT caused side effect are:
- Amnesia
- Confusion
- Palpitation nausea, vomiting
- Dizziness, dry mouth
- Headache
- Fatigue, muscle pain
- Anxiety
- Tongue bite.

Complication:
- Respiratory arrest
- Memory loss
- In direct ECT shoulder, ribs, wrist and other joint fracture may occur.

Q.13. What is ECT failure?

Ans. ECT failure is the condition when tonic clonic convulsion does not occur when current is passed through electrodes it is because of poor physical status, dehydration and overdose of benzodiazepine. To prevent ECT failure hydration must be corrected and improve general physical status of patient.

Q.14. What is prolonged seizure in ECT?

Ans. Seizure continuing beyond 180 second should be considered as prolonged seizures. It must be terminated using fast acting benzodiazepine.

Q.15. Fill ups:

1. __________ is a technique of behavior psychotherapy.
2. __________ is synonymous to therapeutic community.
3. __________ is technique of psychoanalysis.
4. Dose of sodium pentathol in ECT is __________.
5. Succinlylcholine is administered at the rate of __________.

Keys

1. Behavior modification
2. Millieu therapy
3. Free Association
4. 5 mg/kg body weight (150–200 mg)
5. 0.75 mg/kg body weight (30–50 mg)

Q.16. Multiple Choice Questions:

I. ECT is contraindicated in all of these except:
1. Anxiety Neurosis.
2. Fresh Angina Pectoris.
3. Intracranial pressure.
4. All of these.

II. ECT is indicated in following condition:
1. Premorbid personality
2. Early morning insomnia
3. Major depression
4. All of these

III. Following drug is choice of treatment in mania?
1. Phenobarbital
2. Chlorpromazine
3. Librium
4. Lithium carbonate

IV. Following drug is sedative in the barbiturate group of drugs:
1. Haloperidol
2. Pacitan
3. Valium
4. Phenobarbital

V. Which drug is used as antianxiety drug of nonbarbiturate group of drugs?
1. Chlorpromazine
2. Librium
3. Valium
4. Lithium carbonate

VI. Behavior therapy includes all of these except:
1. Cognitive behavior therapy
2. Reciprocal inhibition
3. Systemic modification
4. Assertiveness training
5. All of above

VII. Psychosocial therapy includes all of these except:
1. Psychoanalysis
2. Hypnotherapy
3. Somatic therapy
4. Reality therapy

Keys

Q. I - [4] Q. II - [4] Q. III - [4] Q. IV - [4] Q. V - [2]
Q. VI - [5] Q. VII - [3]

Q.17. Define Psychotherapy. What are the goals of Psychotherapy?

Ans. Psychotherapy is defined by legos as method of treatment based on the development of an intimate (therapeutic) relationship between client/patient and therapist for the purpose of exploring or modifying the patient is behavior in a satisfying direction.

Goals of Psychotherapy:
- Changing maladaptive behavior
- Modifying environment causing maladaptive behavior
- Improving IPR Skill
- Helping the patients to overcome a feeling of handicap
- Helping him to make an accurate assessment of himself and develop self-identity.

Q.18. What are the types of psychotherapy?

Ans.
- Individual psychotherapy
- Behavioural psychotherapy
- Interpersonal psychotherapy
- Group psychotherapy
- Psychosocial therapy

Q.19. What are the techniques used in individual psychotherapy?

Ans.

Psychoanalysis | Hypnosis | Reality therapy | Supportive environmental modification ventilation | In sight psychotherapy | Abreaction

Q.20. Match the following:

A	B
1. Technique to bring internal forces, conflict, childhood trauma and post memories	(a) Insight psychotherapy
2. A technique of relaxation and concentration attention on a single object	(b) Reality therapy
3. A therapeutic technique in which patient talks about repressed emotion by reviving and reliving painful experience	(c) Psychoanalysis
4. A therapy focuses on the present behavior and development of patient's ability to cope with stress of reality	(d) Hypnosis
5. Free expression of feeling or emotion through talk	(e) Abreaction
6. A method of improving well-being of mental patient by changing their living condition	(f) Environmental modification
7. A technique used to modify patient faulty behavior by using his power of reasoning	(g) Reassurance
	(h) Reeducation
	(i) Ventilation
	(j) Assertiveness

Keys

(1) – c (2) – d (3) – d (4) – b
(5) – I (6) – f (7) – h

Q.21. Define Behavior psychotherapy. What are its types?

Ans. Behavior Psychotherapy: "Behavior psychotherapy is a form of psychotherapy which focuses on modifying a faulty behavior rather than basic changes in the personality"

It types are as follows:

- Behavior modification
- Systemic desensitization
- Aversion therapy
- Assertiveness training therapy
- Cognitive behavior therapy
- Implosive therapy (Flooding)
- Positive reinforcement
  - Response shaping
  - Modeling
  - Token economy.

Q.22. Give One Word Answer:

Ans.

1. **A method in which reward or punishment is given to change maladaptive behavior pattern is called.**

Ans. Behavior modification.

2. **Therapy in which there is gradual removal of anxiety or fear is known as**

Ans. Systemic desensitization.

3. **A therapy in which maladaptive or faculty behavior is removed by introducing painful or unpleasant stimuli is termed as**

Ans. Aversion therapy.

4. **Which behavior therapy is useful for depressive patient and for adjustment difficulties?**

Ans. Cognitive behavior therapy.

5. **In which therapy an individual is exposed directly to a maximum intensity fear producing situation to treat phobia**

Ans. Implosive therapy (Flooding)

6. **Therapy in which client is exposed to the ritual behavior such as handwashing and time is limit as to reduce ritualistic behavior is**

Ans. Exposure – response prevention therapy.

7. **Seasonal affective depressive disorder is treated with which therapy**

Ans. Light therapy.

8. **Chronic Sleeplessness is treated with therapy**

Ans. Progressive muscle relaxation

SECTION 3

Pediatric Nursing

- Pediatric

CHAPTER 36

Pediatric

Q.1. What is the clinical problem with preterm babies?

Ans. Clinical problem with preterm babies are:
- Intracranial hemorrhage
- Respiratory distress syndrome
- Infection and feeding problem
- Poor tempreture control
- Necrotising enterocolitis

Q.2. What are retrolental fibroplasias?

Ans. Continuous oxygen therapy in preterm infants leads to blindness due to toxic effects of high blood oxygen concentration on retinal blood vessels. Hence it is essential to ensure that pO_2 does not rise above 90 mm of Hg in preterm babies.

Q.3. What is the prenatal infection?

Ans. Prenatal infections are:
- Septicemia when mother had blood serum infection or placental infection
- AIDS
- Congenital syphilis
- Congenital toxoplasmosis
- Cytomegalic inclusion disease.

Q.4. What is TORCH infection?

Ans.
- Toxoplasma
- Rubella
- Cytomegalovirus
- Herpes simplex

Q.5. What is septicemia?

Ans. Septicemia is invasion and multiplication of organism in bloodstream.

Q.6. What are the causes of septicemia?

Ans. Bloodstream infection with E. coli, Pseudomonas, Klebsiella, Streptococci Listeria and anaerobes are causes of septicemia.

Q.7. What are the features of septicemia in newborn?

Ans. Features of septicemia in newborn are:

- Infants appear grey and apathic
- Refuse to feed with vomiting and diarrhea
- Subnormal temperature
- Splenomegaly and hepatomegaly
- Pyemic abcess

Q.8. Who coined the term kwashiorkor?

Ans. Professor William coined the term kwashiorkor meaning 'red–boy'.

Q.9. What are the clinical features of kwashiorkor?

Ans. Clinical features of kwashiorkor are

- Apathic child with dull looks
- Generalized edema due to hypoalbuminia
- Enlarged liver due to fatty changes
- Skin-hypopigmentation/hyperpigmentation
- Anemia.

Q.10. Which high protein diet is recommended for kwashiorkor child?

Ans. Skimmed milk, soyabean flour and jaggery recommended for kwashiorkor child.

Q.11. What are the features of marasmus?

Ans.
- Wasting of muscles and subcutaneous fat
- Growth retardation.

Q.12. What symptoms are common in both PEM diseases?

Ans. Diarrhea, vitamine deficiency, infection and parasitic infestation are common in both PEM diseases.

Q.13. What are the complications of chikenpox?

Ans. Complication of chickenpox are:

- Bronchopneumonia,
- Herpes zoster,
- Myocarditis,
- Bacterial infection,
- Encephalitis, etc.

Q.14. What is the complication of measles?

Ans. Complication of measles are:

- Bronchiolitis, tracheobronchitis, pneumonia, encephalitis, bleeding diathesis, myocarditis.
- Corneal ulceration.

Q.15. What are the complications of mumps?

Ans.
- Orchitis in boy
- Oophritis in girls
- Meningoencephalitis
- Pancreatitis
- Facial palsy
- Myocarditis

Q.16. What is a whoop?

Ans. A prolonged distressing paroxysm of cough followed by an inspiratory gasp like the crowing sound is called whoop.

Q.17. How will you diagnose whooping cough?

Ans. Typical whoop in infants in young children there will be:

- Lymphocytosis
- Positive fluorescent antibody test
- Positive culture of B Pertussis in Bordet Gengu medium

Q.18. What are the complications of whooping cough?

Ans. Complication of whooping cough are:

- Collapse, pneumothorax,
- Activation of old tuberculosis,
- Epistaxis, subconjunctival hemorrhage and frenular ulcer,
- Rectal prolapsed, inguinal and umbilical hernias.

Q.19. What are the sites for diphtherial infection?

Ans.

- Pharynx
- Tonsils
- Nose
- Skin
- Conjunctiva
- Wound and genitalia.

Q.20. For what Corynebacterium stands for?

Ans. The greek name for the term is korynee-club; bakterion-staff; diphtherion-leather hide; meaning a club shaped bacillus that causes leathery membrane.

Q. 21. What are the complications of diphtheria?

Ans. Myocarditis, peripheral neuritis, bronchopneumonia, cerebral infarction, thrombocytopenia.

Q.22. What are the blood changes in cholera?

Ans.

- Acidosis
- Hypernatremia
- Hypokalemia
- Hypoglycemia

Q.23. What is "coma-vigil"?

Ans. In sever typhoid toxemia, patient lies immobile in a semiconscious state with eyes open and continues to mutter to him, a state known as coma vigil.

Q.24. What are the diagnostic features of tetanus?

Ans. The diagnostic features of tetanus are:

- Lock jaw or trismus
- Stiffness of neck and other muscles, dysphagia, dysphonia and hyperreflexia
- Painful convulsion in an alert patient with a minimal stimulus
- Muscles remain stiff in between the attacks

Q.25. What is pseudotetanus?

Ans. Metoclopramide (perinorm), phenothiazine (phenargan) induced EPS, neuromuscular syndrome is often referred to as pseudotetanus.

Q.26. What are the complications of tetanus?

Ans.

- Laryngospasm with hypoxia
- Aspiration pneumonia

- Venous thrombosis
- Hyperactivity of sympathetic nervous system
- Tachyarrhythmias
- Myocarditis

Q.27. What is treatment for tetanus?

Ans. Treatment for tetanus are:
- Tetanus human immunoglobin 5,000 Ut. IM
- Antitetanus serum 10,000 Ut to older children and 50,000 Ut to young children IV after skin test
- Active immunization with 0.5 ml of T. toxoid 3 doses or booster
- Control of seizures with inj. Diazepam and chlorpromazine
- Inj. procaine penicillin 4 lacs IM daily for 5 days
- Maintenance of nutrition.

Q.28. What is rheumatic fever?

Ans. Rheumatic fever is an inflammatory disease involving heart, joints, CNS, skin, subcutaneous tissues and occurs as delayed sequel to pharyngeal infection with group Streptococci.

Q.29. What is the serological evidenced of recent rheumatic fever?

Ans. ASO Titer more than 150 Ut in adult and more than 333 Ut in children above 5 years.
Antistreptozyme titer more than 200 Ut/ml.

Q.30. What are the diagnostic tests in rheumatic fever?

Ans.
- Antibodies titres are
- Antistreptolysine "O" titre
- AntiDNAse B
- Antistreptozyme test
- Antistreptokinase

Q.31. What is the specific cure for rheumatic fever?

Ans. There is no specific cure for rheumatic fever and no known measures change the course of an attack good supportive therapy only reduces the morbidity and mortality.

Q.32. What are the measures for rheumatic fever prophylaxis?

Ans. Inj. Benzathine penicilline-1.2 mega Ut IM at 3 to 4 week interval

Or

Sulphadizine 0.5 gm once daily for those below 60 Ib 1 gm daily for those above 60 Ib

Or

Oral penicilline 2,00000 Ut twice daily

Or

Erythromycine 250 mg twice daily

The therapy should continue for life

Q.33. What are the causes of congestive cardiac failure in the newborn?

Ans.
- Transposition of great vessels
- Hypoplastic left heart syndrome

- Double outlet right ventricle without pulmonary stenosis
- Arotic atresia and aortic arch interruption
- Aortic pulmonary window large patent ductus arterious (PDA)
- Right pulmonary stenosis or atresia

Q.34. What are the features of congestive heart failure?

Ans.
- Anorexia
- Dispropotionate tachycardia
- Raised JVP
- Peripheral cyanosis
- Hepatomegaly
- Bilateral piting edema.

Q.35. What do you mean by unhealthy tonsils?

Ans.
- Unhealthy tonsils indicates
- Chronically hypertrophied tonsils covered with slough
- Enlarged jugulodigastric and cervical lymph nodes
- Poor appetite, failure to gain weight, etc.

Q.36. When will you advice tonsillectomy?

Ans. Chronic tonsillitis that causes retarded growth and development of child and frequent upper respiratory infection. Retrotonsillar abscess.

Q.37. Why stridor persisting after birth?

Ans. Larngeomalacia and tracheomalacia that lead to flabbiness of supraglottic aperture and weakness of airway walls leading to collapse and airway obstruction during inspiration.

Q.38. What is hyaline membrane disease?

Ans. Deficient synthesis and degradation or functional alteration in surfactant and a complaint chest wall in small infants lead to idiopathic respiratory distress syndrome characterized by- Effusion of a proteinacious material into alveolar spaces with hypoxia and features of respiratory failure.

Q.39. What are the pathological changes in hyaline membrane disease?

Ans. The lungs are liver like in consistency. Microscopically there is atelectasis is with engorgement of interalveolar capillaries and lymphatics. An acidophilic homogenous granular membrane lines the alveolar and small bronchioles interalveolar hemorrhage and interstitial emphysema may be found.

Q.40. How will you suspect hyaline membrane disease?

Ans. Respiratory distress characterized by:
- Rapid shallow respiration
- Grunting intercostals and subcostal retraction
- Cyanosis unresponsive to oxygen administration
- Progressive air hunger
- Dull percussion.

Q.41. What is primary complex?

Ans. A subpleural Ghon's focus, usually a centimeter in diameter together with prominent lymphatics channels and enlarged lymph nodes draining the area constitute the primary complex.

Q.42. When would you suspect primary complex?

Ans. Suspect primary complex when:

- Failure to gain weight
- Anorexia
- Mild irregular fever
- Occasional cough
- Vague ill health

Q.43. What is mantoux test?

Ans. Mantoux test is an intradermal skin test to know if a person has developed hypersensitivity to tubercle bacilli.

Q.44. How mantoux test helps in clinical diagnosis?

Ans. A strongly positive more than 15 × 15 mm induration indicates ongoing tuberculosis process.

Q.45. What are the bactericidal antituberculous drugs?

Ans. Streptomycine, caprecomycine, cycloserine,

- INH
- Rifampicine
- Pyrazinamide.

Q.46. What are side effects of INH?

Ans. Direct toxic effects like polyneuropathy, anemia.

- Allergic reaction in the form of skin rash, swelling of tongue, arthralgia and fever
- Hepatitis caused by INH degradation products in the liver.

Q.47. What are the side effects of rifampicine?

Ans.
- Hypersensitivity reaction like flu syndrome
- Fever, gastrointestinal symptoms, hepatitis.

Q.48. What precaution should you take for ethambutol therapy?

Ans. Ethambutol causes optic neuritis, children below 5 year in whom visual acuity cannot be followed should not be prescribed ethambutol. Older children taking ethambutol should undergo periodic evaluation of visual acuity, perimetry and color vision testing.

Q.49. What is protinuria?

Ans. Daily urinary protein excreation more than 150 mg.

Q.50. What is the source of protein found in normal urine?

Ans. Tamm-Horsefall mucoprotien, an alfa globulin of high molecular weight formed in the kidneys.

Globulines formed in urinary tract and seminal vesicles.

Q.51. What are causes of pyuria?

Ans. Infection with tuberculosis, fungi, mycobacteria anaerobes, Hemophilus influenzae.

Urinary tract calculus: papillary necrosis of any cause.

Renal infiltration with myeloma or lymphoma.

Q.52. Why you see broad casts in CRF?

Ans. The broad casts reflect compensatory dilatation hypertrophy of surviving nephrons.

Q.53. What are the causes of hematuria in children?

Ans.
- Hereditary renal disorder
- Hereditary nephritis with deafness
- Familial benign recurrent hematuria
- Polycystic kidney

Glomerulonephritis
- Acute post streptococcal
- Membranoproliferative
- Berger's IgA and IgG disease
- Wilm's tumor
- Bacterial endocarditis
- Nephrolithiasis
- Urinary tract infection
- Coagulation disorder.

Q.54. What are the salt wasting nephropathies?

Ans.
- Chronic pyelonephritis.
- Polycystic and medullary cystic diseases.
- Tuble interstitial diseases that include renal injury due analgesics, lead, antibiotics, heavy metals, uric acid, hypercalcemia, leukemias.

Q.55. What are the causes of polyuria?

Ans.
- Diabetes mellitus
- Diabetes insipidus
- Chronic renal failure
- Hypokalemia.

Q.56. What are the functions of kidneys?

Ans.
- Excretion of metabolic waste
- Synthesis of 1-25 dihydroxy vit D3
- Secretion of erythropoietin and renin.

Q.57. When will you subject a child for intravenous pyelography?

Ans.
- Abdominal mass
- Abnormal genitalia
- Urinary tract infection
- Neurogenic bladder
- Unexplained renal failure
- Hypertension
- Nephrolithiasis

Q.58. What are the indications for renal angiography?

Ans.
- Hypertension where renal artery stenosis, fibro plasia or anomaly are suspected.
- Renal trauma where IVP does not visualize the kidney or there is marked extravasation of the dye.

Q.59. What are the causes of bilateral enlargement of kidneys with CRF?

Ans.
- Polycystic disease.
- Renal involvement in diabetes, SLE, amyloidosis
- Renal vein thrombosis
- Hypersensitive nephropathy

Q.60. What are the causes of renal failure?

Ans. Pre renal causes:
- Hypovolemia due to external/internal blood loss, extensive burns, pancreatitis, peritonitis.
- Cardiac failure due to extensive infarction, tamponade.

Renal causes
- Glomerulonephritis.
- Interstitial nephritis.
- Vascular diseases like vasculitis due to DIC, TTP. Hemolytic uraemic syndrome, malignant hypertension arterial or venous occlusion, hepatorenal syndrome.
- Acute tubular necrosis due to all renal causes as above, hemolytic transfusion reactions, rhabdomyolysis, contrast material reactions.
- Renal vein thrombosis.

Postrenal causes
- Obstruction to ureters due to clots, stone, necrosed papillae, retroperitoneal fibrosis.
- Renal vein thrombosis.

Q.61. What is non oliguric renal failure?

Ans. This is less sever form of renal failure with GFR 5 to 10 ml/min and daily urine output between 500 and 1000 ml.

Q.62. What are the causes of nonoliguric renal failure?

Ans. Hypovolemia, septic shock, radiographic contrast material, crush injury, etc.

Q.63. What are causes of renal failure in newborn infant?

Ans. Perirenal anoxias, respiratory distress syndrome, sever hemorrhage either maternal or neonatal, septicemia, DIC, hemolytic uremic syndrome, congenital structural anomaly of urinary tract.

Q.64. What are the causes of common causes of chronic renal failure in children?

Ans. Congenital renal and urinary tract malformations, glomerulonephritis, hereditary renal disease, hemolytic uremic syndrome, renal vein thrombosis.

Q.65. What do you mean by rapidly progressive glomerulonephritis (RPGN)?

Ans. RPGN is any glomerular disease in which there is rapid loss of renal function with extensive crescent formation in over 50% glomeruli.

Q.66. What are the causes for rapidly progressive glomerulonephritis?

Ans. Anti GBM
- Antibody mediated
- Good pasteur's syndrome
- Idiopathic anti GBM nephritis
- Associated with granular immune deposits
- Post streptococcal

- SLE
- Henoch-Schonlein purpura
- Cryoglobulinemia
- Membrane proliferative glomerulonephritis
- Idiopathic immune complex disease
- Vasculitis of polyarteritis and Wegener's granulomatosis.

Q.67. What are the immunopathogenetic mechanisms for renal injury?

Ans.
- Anti-tissue antibody mediated disease.
- Antibasement membrane antibody disease.
- Non basement membrane related anti-tissue antibody.
- Immune complex mediated renal disease
- Complement associated renal injury
- Cell mediated immunity response.

Q.68. Why plasma albumin is depressed in nephrotic syndrome?

Ans.
- Excessive urinary loss
- Increased renal catabolism
- Inadequate hepatic synthesis.

Q.69. What are the causes of nephrotic syndrome?

Ans.
- Minimal change disease-70 to 80 percent
- Meangial proliferative GMN-10–15%
- Focal and segmental glomerulosclerosis
- Membranous glomerulopath (rare)
- Membrano proliferative GMN 5–10%
- Infections like syphilis, malaria, filarial, leprosy and hepatitis
- Infectious mononucleosis, schistosmiasis
- Reaction to drugs like penicillamine, captopril, antitoxin
- Multisystem disease like SLE, amyloidosis, sarcoidosis
- Diabetes mellitus, fabry's disease
- Congenital nephritic syndrome.

Q.70. What is the reason for edema in nephritic syndrome?

Ans. Hypoalbuminemia with antecedent decrease in plasmaoncotic pressure leads to disturbance in starling forces acting across peripheral capillaries. Fluid from intravascular compartment shifts to the interstitial tissue. This results information of edema and deficit in effective plasma volume. The latter activates rennin-angiotensin-aldosterone system, enhances secretion of antidiuretic hormone and sympathetic nervous system activity and reduces secretion of natriuretic hormone. All these changes lead to increased absorption of water and salt in distal segments of renal tubules and compound the edema formation.

Q.71. What is the cause of hyperlipidemia in nephrotic syndrome?

Ans.
- Diminished plasma oncotic pressure stimulates hepatic lipoprotein synthesis.
- Excessive urinary excretion of plasma protein factors regulating lipoprotein synthesis or removal.

Q.72. What is the pathology in minimal change disease?

Ans. Diffuse epithelial cell foot process effacement and fusion. No deposits, no proliferative element.

Q.73. How will you dignose Wilm's tumor?

Ans. Renal mass, firm smooth mass, non-tender in a child below 2 yrs is most likely to be Wilm's tumors.

Q.74. What are the differential diagnosis of Wilm's tumors?

Ans. Neuroblastoma, polycystic disease, hydronephrosis, solitary cyst can be differential diagnosis of Wilm's tumors.

Q.75. What is Bartter syndrome?

Ans. It is functional disorder of kidneys .characterized by renal potassium wasting, elevated plasma, renin and aldosterone and hyperplasia of juxtaglomerular apparatus. The blood pressure is normal due to elevated production of renal vasodilator prostaglandins by juxtaglomerular cells.

Q.76. What are the types of calcification in a growth?

Ans.
- Punctuate
- Circumlinear
- Curvelinear
- Popcorn

Q.77. What is the clinical presentation of Wilm's tumor?

Ans.
- Unilateral flank mass, firm, non-tender
- Raised blood pressure due to compression of renal artery by the mass
- Hematuria, weight loss and pain in late cases
- X-ray abdomen shows displacement of intestinal gas shadow and obliteration of psoas shadow on that side

Q.78. What are the causes of repeated urinary tract infection in small children?

Ans.
- Vescicoureteric reflux
- Posterior urethral valves.

Q.79. What is hemolytic uremic syndrome?

Ans. It is charecterised by microangiopathic, Coombs, negative hemolytic anemia, nephropathy AS and thrombocytopenia following a prodromal illness involving gastrointestinal tract or a flu syndrome.

Q.80. Define anemia What is its type?

Ans. Anemia is defined as reduction in red blood cell below normal level or in the concentration of hemoglobulin
- It is classify according to cause
- Decrease production of RBC: iron deficiency anemia
- Hemolytic anemia: Thalassemia
- Hemorrhagic anemia: Accidental, loss of blood, etc.

Fill ups

1. A hereditary bleeding disorder is ____________ (Hemophilia).
2. Prolonged Clotting Time is seen in ____________ (Hemophillia).
3. Shape of RBC in sickle cell anemia is ____________ (sickle shaped).
4. Clinical manifestation of sickle cell anemia developed in the newborn at the age of ____________ (3 to 6 month of age).

5. Uncontrolled abnormal production of WBC is seen in ________ (Leukemia).
6. Hemophilia is developed due to deficiency of ________ (viii, ix, xi). (Clotting factors)
7. Fetal Hb is replaced by adult Hb is ________ (At 6 month of age.)
8. A child with thalassemia should infused with ________ (Washed RBC).
9. The normal blood volume in newborn is ________ (300 cc).
10. An infant begins to sit with support by which months ________ (7 Months).
11. Head control is possible in an infant at ________ (3 months).
12. A child starts crawling at ________ (11 months).
13. Child give social smile at the age of ________ (4 months).
14. First permanent tooth which erupts is ________ (Ist premolar).
15. Number of deciduous teeth is ________ (20).
16. A child starts taking self-decision at age of ________ (6 years).
17. Child changes rattle from one hand to another at the age of ________ (6 months).
18. Vocabulary of 1.5 years old child is ________ (20 words).
19. By ________ years all milk teeth are erupted. (2 years).
20. In Indian babies, normal weight at the time of birth is ________ (2.5 to 3.8 kg).
21. An infant weight is doubled of birth weight by the age of ________ (6 months).
22. At birth an average length of a healthy Indian new born baby is ________ (50 cm).
23. At birth an average head circumference is measured about ________ (35 cm).
24. Posterior fontanell get closed by the age of ________ (6 to 8 weeks).
25. Anterior fontanelle normally gets closed by ________ (12 to 18 months).

Q.81. What is normal hemoglobulin level in children at various ages?

Ans.

Cord blood	16.8 gm%
2 weeks	16.5%
3 month	12 gm%
6 month to 6 year	12 gm%
7 to 12 year	13 gm%

Q.82. What is fetal hemoglobulin?

Ans. Fetal hemoglobulin (HbF) contains two alpha and two gamma chains represented by a2 y2. Its production starts frome 8th weeks of intrauterine life and by 24th weeks it constitutes 90 % of total Hb.

Q.83. What are sideroblastic anemias?

Ans. Sideroblastic anemias are:

- Hereditary or congenital
- Idiopatic
- Associated with leukemias, Hodgkin's disease, myloproliferative disorder

- Drug induced INH, lead poisioning
- They present hypochromic anemia with increased serum iron and ferritin
- Ring sideroblast can be detected in marrow to constitute more than 10% of nuecleated red cells

Q.84. What is the treatment of sideroblastic anemia?

Ans. The treatment of sideroblastic anemia are:

- Pyriodoxamine 200 mg daily
- Trial of androgens
- Transfusion and desferoxamine.

Q.85. What are the effects of anemia on heart?

Ans. The effects of anemia on heart maybe sinus tachycardia, congestive cardiac failure, and angina pectoris.

Q.86. What is the indication of parenteral iron therapy?

Ans.
- Unable to tolerate oral iron
- Blood loss at too rapid rate not to be compensated by oral iron
- Malabsorption syndromes and intestinal disease.

Q.87. How will you calculate total injectable iron?

Ans. Iron to be injected = (patient's Hb in gm/dl) x kg body weight x 3

Q.88. What are the causes of folate deficiency?

Ans.
- Malabsorption syndrome
- Increased requirement of infancy
- Concurrent malignancy
- Antiepileptic drugs like phentoine and barbiturates.

Q.89. Why there is anemia in chronic renal failure?

Ans.
- Diminished secretion of erythropoitin
- Suppression of erythropoiesis by uremia
- Impaired incorporation of iron into developing red cell
- Hemorrhage
- Loss of folic acid during dialysis.

Q.90. What is the effect of sickling?

Ans. The sickle cells are rigid increase blood viscosity. As a result some obstruction to capillary flow is rule and tissue hypoxia results which compounds sickling. These rigid cells when pass through the spleen from circulation and are destroyed.

Q.91. What are the clinical manifestations of sickle cell anemia?

Ans.
- Impaired growth and development
- Incresed susceptibility to infection
- Vaso occlusive crisis
- Anemia.

Q.92. What are the factors affecting sickling?

Ans. Acidosis and increased red cell 2–3 DPG lower oxygen affinity, promote intracellular polymerization and sickling.

- Sickling is dependent upon HbS concentration.

- Red cell dehydration due to hypertonic environment as in renal medulla also increases sickling. Hence papillary renal infarcts is common in SS or even AS disease.

Q.93. Which factors are responsible for aplastic crisis in sickle cell disease?

Ans.
- Infection
- Folic acid deficiency

Q.94. What will be the skeletal changes occurred in sickle cell disease?

Ans.
- Biconcave fish mouth vertebra.
- Aseptic necrosis of femoral head.
- Frequent Salmonella osteomyelitis superimposed upon bone infarction.

Q.95. What are the causes of recurrent acute abdominal pain in children?

Ans.
- Worm infestation
- Porphyria
- Intussusceptions
- Meckel's diverticulitis
- Lead poisoning
- Crisis of diabetes
- Sickle cell disease
- Typhlitis
- Abdominal angina

Q.96. What is sickling test?

Ans. RBCs show sickling in sickle cell disease when the oxygen tension is reduced by-
1. Addition of meta bisulfate.
2. Incubated in a covered slide for 24 hours.

Q.97. What is methemoglobin?

Ans. Normally the Hb iron is in reduced form (Fe^{2+}). When it is oxidized it becomes Fe^{3+} and is devoid of oxygen carrying capacity commonly termed as methemoglobin.

Q.98. What are the acquired causes of methemoglobinemia?

Ans. Administration of drugs like amylnitrite, nitroprusside, phenacetin, lidocaine, etc. is the acquired causes of methemoglobinemia.

Q.99. What are the clinical manifestations of methemoglobinemia?

Ans. If patient showing cyanosis without evidence of clinical lung or heart disease are the clinical manifestations of methemoglobinemia.

Q.100. What are thalassemias?

Ans. Thalassemias are a group of congenital disorders in which there is defective synthesis in the globin units. So strictly speaking they are not hemoglobinopathies as here is only quantitative abnormality in globin synthesis whereas in the former the quality of Hb is defective.

Q.101. What are the characteristic features of beta thalassemia major?

Ans.
- Infective erythropoiesis
- Extramedullary hematopoiesis with enlarged liver and spleen
- Shortened RBC life span
- Bone marrow hyperplasia.

Q.102. What will be the characteristic X-ray features of bone marrow hyperplasia in thalassemia major?

Ans.
- Enlarged molar bones.
- Hair on end appearance of skull bones.
- Para vertebral masses.
- Enlarged medullary cavity of metacarpals.

Q.103. What are the treatments for beta thalassemia major?

Ans. The treatment for beta thalassemia major are as follows:
- Frequent blood transfusion to keep hemoglobin above 7 gm percent
- Folic acid supplement
- Desferoxamine to prevent hemosiderosis
- Genetic counseling
- Prenatal diagnosis and therapeutic abortion.

Q.104. What is congenital aplastic anemia?

Ans. It is associated with multiple congenital anomalies and chromosomal abnormality. They have a high-risk of developing leukemia.

Q.105. What are the indications for marrow transplantation?

Ans.
- Immunologic deficient diseases.
- Aplastic anemias.
- Acute leukemias and selected cases of chronic leukemias.

Q.106. What are the complications of bone marrow transplantation?

Ans.
- Acute graft vs host disease
- Chronic graft vs host disease
- Marrow graft rejection

Q.107. What are causes of thrombocytopenia?

Ans.
- Production defect
- Reduced thrombosis in marrow invasion or aplasia
- Defective maturation in B12, folic acid deficiency
- Increased sequestration in splenomegaly
- Accelerated destruction due to auto antibodies and allo-antibodies
- Excessive consumption as in TTP and DIC

Q.108. What are the features of thrombocytopenia?

Ans. Spontaneous bleeding into skin and mucous membranes manifesting as ecchymosis and blood filled bullae in oral cavity are the features of thrombocytopenia.

Q.109. What is thrombocythemia?

Ans. Sustained elevation of platelet count beyond 8,00,000/cubic mm in polycythemia vera, chronic myeloid leukemia and myelosclerosis is termed thrombocythemia.

Q.110. What is hemophilia?

Ans. It is a coagulation disorder due to inherited deficiency in procoagulant activity of factor VIII.

Q.111. What is the function of antihemophilic factor?

Ans. It acts as a cofactor for factor IX in the activation of factor X.

Q.112. How will you diagnose hemophilia?

Ans. If family history of bleeding tendency affecting only males.

- Normal prothrombin time
- Prolonged partial thromboplastin time
- Reduced to absent VIII coagulant antigen in blood.

Q.113. Which analgesics are safe to be used by hemophiliacs?

Ans.
- Propoxyphene
- Paracetamol.

Q.114. What is disseminated intravascular coagulation (DIC)?

Ans. It is a syndrome characterized by liberation of thrombin in circulation with consumption of platelets and coagulation factors which ultimately lead to bleeding tendency.

Q.115. How will you diagnose DIC?

Ans.
- Thrombocytopenia
- Hypofibrinogenemia and increased fibrinogen degradation products
- Elevated fibrinopeptide A and fibrin monomer
- Prolonged prothrombin and partial thromboplastin time.

Q.116. What do you understand by polycythemia rubra vera?

Ans. It is a combination of polycythemia, leukocytes thrombocytosis, splenomegaly and hyperplastic bone marrow.

Q.117. What are the tests to diagnose G6PD deficiency?

Ans.
- Methemoglobin dye reduction test
- G6PD bioassay.

Q.118. Which drugs are likely to produce hemolysis in G6PD deficient patients?

Ans.
- Primaquine
- Aspirin
- PAS
- Chloramphenicol
- Vit K
- Sulphas
- Nitrofurans
- Choloquine, quinine.

Q.119. What is the nursing intervention to relive bone pain in Thalassemia?

Ans. Monitor CBC, if less than 10 gm reported to the consultant
- Elevate lower extremities
- Apply warm bath or soaks
- Administer NSAIDS like ibrufen
- Monitor LFT.

Q.120. What are the nursing interventions to control bleeding in hemophilia?

Ans. Apply cold and pressure over the area (immediately after IV/IM injection).
- Place fibrin foam on the wound
- Avoid suturing
- Avoid fast administration of IP Drugs
- Avoid rectal temperature
- Check toys for rough edges
- Do not give hard candy and sharp utensils.

Q.121. What is hyperbilirubinemia?

Ans. It is an elevated level of bilirubine in the blood.

Q.122. What causes hyperbilirubinemia?

Ans.
- Faster breakdown of RBC
- Decrease removal of bilirubine by the liver
- It can be because of physiologic, hemolytic and sepsis.

Q.123. When bilirubine dangerous to brain?

Ans. A more than 20 mg% of bilirubine is dangerous to brain.

Q.124. What are the treatments in hyperbilirubinemia?

Ans.
- Phototherapy–fluorescent light
- Exchange transfusion.

Q.125. What are the nursing cares to be followed for baby in phototherapy?

Ans.
- Undressed the baby
- Cover the eye
- Put the nappy over the genitalia
- Maintained hydration
- Avoid overheating to baby
- Prevent cross infection.

Q.126. What are the dangers of phototherapy?

Ans. The danger of phototherapy can be:
- Eye damage
- Eye patches may develop and may obstruct nasal breathing
- Increased water loss through evaporation.

Q.127. What are the indications of splenectomy?

Ans.
- Hereditary spherocytosis,
- Hypersplenism,
- Warm antibody autoimmune hemolytic anemia.

Q.128. What are the features of tumor lysis syndrome?

Ans.
- Hyperuremia, uratenephropathy
- Hyperphosphtemia
- Hyperkalemia-cardiac arrest.

Q.129. Which congenital disease must be excluded soon after birth?

Ans.
- Esophageal atresia
- Tacho-esophageal cleft
- Cricopharyngeal dysfunction

Q.130. What is atypical febrile convulsion?

Ans. Convulsion that occur at normal or nearly normal temperature, last for more than 20 minutes is focal and abnormal ECG changes seen.

Q.131. What are the causes of microcephaly?

Ans. Defects in brain development as in mongolism and other autosomal and trisomy disorder, ionizing radiation.
- Dwarfism
- Intrauterine TORCH infection
- Intrauterine anoxia, neonatal hypoxia, severe malnutrition in early infancy

Q.132. What are the common etiologic agents of pyogenic meningitis in small children?

Ans. The common etiologic agents of pyogenic meningitis in small children are–

- H. Influenzae
- Pneumococci
- Meningococci
- Staphylococci
- Streptococci
- E. Coli Listeria.

Q.133. What are the complications of meningitis?

Ans.
- Encephalitis and brain abscess
- Basal meningitis with cranial nerve palsy and hydrocephalus
- Subdural effusion
- Cranial thrombophlebitis.

Q.134. What is encopresis?

Ans. It is a condition in which watery colonic content percolate around the hard colonic fecal masses in constipating children and pass per rectum without childs awareness.

Q.135. Which the congenital diseases must be excluded soon after the birth?

Ans.
- Esophageal atresia
- Tacho-esophageal cleft and fistula
- Imperforated anus
- Congenital anomalis of urethra.

Q.136. What are neuromuscular disorders that may cause dysphagia?

Ans.
- Cerebral palsy
- Cranial nerve palsy
- Acalasia
- Motility disorder of esophagus
- Muscular dystrophy
- Scleroderma.

Q.137. What is the feature of congenital pyloric stenosis?

Ans.
- Projectile vomiting 2 to 3 weeks after birth
- Visible peristalsis moving from left to right
- Hard mobile, painless mass in right upper quadrant, best palpable after the child has vomited.

Q.138. How is congenital duodenal obstruction diagnosed?

Ans.
- Billious vomiting soon after birth
- Dobble bubble gas shadow one above the other in plain X-ray abdomen in upright position
- No gas in the intestine if obstruction is complete.

Q.139. What are the causes of viral diarrheas in children?

Ans.
- Rotavirus infection
- Norwalk viruses
- Enteroviruses
- Acute exanthema like measles, influenza virus.

Q.140. What are the features of viral diarrheas?

Ans.
- Vomiting precedes diarrhea
- Green offensive stool contains mucus and milk curds
- Mild fever and dehydration in proportion to intensity of diarrhea.

Q.141. What are the features of dehydration of in small children?

Ans. Loss of skin turgor and elasticity
- Irritability, drowsiness, lethargy
- Sunken eyes, depressed fontanelle, dry lips and tongue
- Oliguria, hypotension, rapid thredy pulse
- Weight loss more than 10% in severe diarrhea.

Q.142. How will you plan fluid therapy in mild to moderate diarrhea?

Ans. ORS is preferred; 50 ml of ORS /kg to be taken within 4 to 5 hours for mild dehydration and 100 ml of ORS/kg 4 hours for moderate dehydration.

Q.143. What are causes of bacterial diarrheas in children?

Ans. E. coli, Shigella, Salmonella, Vibrio, Clostridium, Staphylococci.

Q.144. What is the line of treatment of diarrhea?

Ans.
- Prompt rehydration and fluid supplement for ongoing losses
- Rest to GI tract
- Symtomatic relief with antimotility agent and astringents.

Q.145. What are the antimotility agents used in diarrhea?

Ans.
- Lomotil 0.25 mg/kg/day in divided dose
- Loperamide 0.1 mg/kg/for 2–3 doses
- Codeinophos 1 mg/kg/day in divided doses.

Q.146. What are the causes of noninfective diarrhea in children?

Ans.
- Food allergy
- Food poisioning
- Overfeeding.
- Antibiotic induced, intestinal worm, disaccharidase deficiency.

Q.147. What are the WHO formulas for ORS?

Ans.
- Sodium chloride 3.5 gm
- Sodium bicarbonate 2.5 gm
- Potassium chloride 1.5 gm
- Glucose 25 gm.

Q.148. How will you define chronic diarrhea?

Ans. Diarrhea of at least 3 weeks duration or 3 attacks of diarrhea during 3 months.

Q.149. What is cow's milk allergy?

Ans. Introduction of cow's milk in infants causes: Diarrhea, vomiting, colic, urticaria, eczema, rhinitis, cough, wheeze that is caused by presense of betalactoglobulin in cow's milk.

Q.150. What is Wilson's disease?

Ans. Wilson's disease is an autosomal recessive disorder of copper metabolism that leads to excessive accumulation of copper in brain, liver and kidney.

Q.151. What are the clinical symptoms of Wilson's disease?

Ans.
- Hepatomegaly often with cirrhosis
- EPS with mental disorder
- Coombs negative hemolytic anemia
- Fanconi syndrome and CRF
- Amenorrhea/repeated abortion.

Q.152. What is the treatment of Wilson's disease?

Ans.
- D-penicillamine 20 mg/kg in 4 divided doses before meals and at bedtime with vit B6.
- Triethylene tetramine or dimarcaprol if patient intolerant to penicillamine.

Q.153. What are the causes of convulsion in childhood?

Ans. Before 1 month Birth injury, hypoxia, phenylketonuria, hypoglycemia, kernicterus, TORCH, Congenital abnormalities of brain and CNS infection.
- 1 to 6 months: CNS infection, head injury, TB, cerebral malaria, malformation, drugs.
- 6 months to 3 year febrile convulsion and above all mentioned.
- 3 years to 12 years: Idiopathic epilepsy.

Q.154. What is febrile convulsion?

Ans. Generalized seizure occurring between 6 months to 3 years of age when body temperature cross 38° C is called febrile convulsion. The attack last for less than 20 minutes. No ECG, EEG Changes occur.

Q.155. What is the treatment of meningitis?

Ans.
- Ampicilline 100 mg/kg/I.V. in 4 in divided doses.

OR

- Chloramhenicol 50 to 100 mg/kg/IV in 4 divided doses
- Penicilline + chloramphenicol as in adults may be given to older children
- Anti-edema measure and other supportive.

Q.156. What are the stages of TB meningitis?

Ans. **Prodormal stage:** Apathy, irritability, headache, mild fever, intellectual deterioration

Transitional stage: Manisfestation as meningeal irritation and raised ICP

Terminal stage: paralysis, coma.

Q.157. What are the complications of TB meningitis?

Ans.
- Mental retardation
- Hydrocephalus
- Cranial nerve palsy
- Spastic hemiplegia, atexia, diabetes other endocrinal disturbance.

Q.158. What are the treatments for TB meningitis?

Ans.
- Anti tubercular therapy
- Rifampicine 10 to 20 mg/kg/day single dose for 18 to 24 month along with INH 20 mg/day single dose
- Streptomycine 40 to 50 mg/kg/IM/for initial 3 months
- Anti edema measures
- Prednisone 1 to 2 mg/kg/day/for 1 to 3 months.

Q.159. What are the problems with postterm babies?

Ans. Postterm or LGA (Large gestational age) babies have some typical problem like:
- Asphyxia
- RDS
- Hypoglycemia, etc.

Q.160. What is Hyperthermia?

Ans. An elevated or higher than a normal temperature (37° C) of newborn is called as hyperthermia.

Q.161. What are the causes of hyperthermia?

Ans.
- Sepsis (infection)
- Dehydration
- Enviormental–phototherapy, over wrapping.

Q.162. What are the clinical problems with hyperthermia?

Ans.
- Tachycardia, tachypnea
- Poor feeding
- Decreased activity
- Weak cry, apnea, hypotension sweating, etc.

Q.163. What is hypothermia? What are causes of hypothermia?

Ans. A lower than normal temperature is called hypothermia. The main reasons are blood infection, heat loss.

Q.164. What are the signs and symptoms of hypothermia?

Ans.
- Cyanosis
- Pallor
- Cool extremities
- Lethargic
- Apnea bradycardia
- Poor feeding.

Q.165. What are the complications of hypothermia?

Ans.
- Hypoglycemia
- Acidosis
- Hypoxia

Q.166. Multiple choice questions.

1. **Baby friendly hospital concept was launced by WHO in the year**
   (a) 1997 (b) 1991
   (c) 1999 (d) 2001
2. **In India baby friendly hospital concept was launched in year**
   (a) 1987 (b) 1994
   (c) 1992 (d) 1995
3. **WHO launched global immunization program in which year?**
   (a) 1970 (b) 1972
   (c) 1979 (d) 1974
4. **Which are the triple vaccine?**
   (a) Oral Polio (b) BCG
   (c) DPT (d) Rabies

5. Which is killed vaccine?

(a) BCG (b) Pertussis
(c) Oral Polio (d) Mumps

6. MMR should be given at which months.

(a) 6 month (b) 9 month
(c) 12 month (d) 18 month

Keys

(1) – b (2) – c (3) – d (4) – c
(5) – b (6) – d

Q.167. Fill ups:

1. The rout for BCG vaccination is __________. (intradermal)
2. OPV vaccine is best stored at __________ degree centigrade temperature. (2–10°)
3. The route for triple vaccine administrations is __________. (intramuscular)
4. Contraindication for DPT vaccination is __________. (progressive neurogical disease)
5. The dose of rubella vaccine is __________. (0.5 ml)

Q.168. Define Play.

Ans. "Play is an instinctive preparation for adulthood" it is business of childhood.

Q.169. What are the value of play?

Ans.
- Physical development
- Intellectual development
- Creative
- Therapeutic
- Socialization.

Q.170. What are the stages of play in children?

Ans.
1. Exploratory stage (3–12 months)
2. Toy stage (1-6-8 years)
3. Play stage
4. Day dreaming stage.

Q.171. What are the purpose of baby friendly hospital?

Ans.
- Improved antenatal care
- Mother friendly delivery services
- Immunication
- Diarrhea management
- Providing good nutrition and promotion of health growth
- Wide spread availability of family planning.

Q.172. Define Immunization.

Ans. It is a process of protecting an individual from diseases through introduction of line of killed or attenuated organism in the individuals body. It prevents pediatric population from mortality morbidity and handicapped condition.

Q.173. Define Vaccine.

Ans. Vaccines are immuno-biological substances which produces specific protection against a given disease it stimulates production of antibodies.

Q.174. Define cold chain. What are the cold chain equipment?

Ans. The 'cold chain' is a system of storing and transporting vaccines at low temperature from the manufactures to the actual vaccination location so that their potency and efficacy are presolved cold chain equipments are:

- Cold box
- Vaccine carrier
- Flask
- Ice pack
- Refrigerator/Freezer.

Q.175. Match the following:

Ans.

A	B
1. Triple vaccine	(a) EPI
2. Tuberculosis	(b) Under five clinic
3. Tetanus toxoid	(c) Baby friendly hospital
4. Family planning	(d) Cold chain
5. WHO	(e) DPT
6. Cold box	(f) BCG
7. 10 steps of breastfeeding	(g) Pregnancy

Keys

1 – E, 2 – F, 3 – G, 4 – B, 5 – A, 6 – D, 7 – C

Q.176. What are the common accidental injuries in children?

Ans. Fall, Foreign body aspiration, burns, foreign bodies in ear, nose and mouth, drawing road traffic accidents.

Q.177. What instruction will you give to parents to avoid common hazards and injuries in children?

Ans.

- Instruct about proper storage of poisonous substances
- Instruct to put label on the container
- Poisonous substances should never be placed in container used for the food
- Instruct to seek medical advice when poisonous substance is suspected.

Q.178. What is midday meal program?

Ans. The midday meal program is also known as school lunch program. This program has been in operation since 1961 throughout the country. The major objectives of this program is to attract more and more children for admission to school, so, that literacy of children could be brought about good level of improvement.

Q.179. What do you mean by Down syndrome?

Ans. It is commonest chromosomal abnormality it was first described by Down in 1866 it is also known as trisomy 21.

Q.180. What are the features of Down syndrome?

Ans. Children with Down syndrome have features of:

- Flat face
- Small nose
- Small ears
- Short neck

- Short digits
- Single and palmer creases in hand
- Soft and spores hair
- Dry skin, septal defect

Small genitalia and infertility in males duodenal atresia, oesophageal atresia lymphoplastic leukemia can occur.

Q.181. What are the clinical manifestation of Klinefelter's Syndrome.

Ans. These children present tall stature, poor musculature small testis, delayed puberty, gynecomastia, infertile behavioral and emotional problems.

Q.182. Define genetic counseling.

Ans. According American Society of human "genetics" counseling is a communication process which deals with occurrence or risk of genetic disorder in family.

Q.183. Fill ups:

1. The portion of chromosome which codes for a "Character" is called ________.
2. Arrangement of chromosome in the cell is called ________.
3. Trisomy 21 was first described by ________.
4. The first famous clone born in ________ and Named ________ (a sheep).
5. The total number of chromosome is ________.
6. The genetic make-up of a person is called as ________.
7. Down's syndrome is also known as ________.
8. A male person affected with klienfelter's syndrome have ________ X chromosome and ________ Y chromosome.
9. The position of gene an a chromosome is called ________.
10. Trisomy 13 is also called as ________.

Keys

1. Gene, 2. Karyotype, 3. Down in 1866, 4. 1997 dolly, 5. 46, 6. Genotype, 7. Mongolism, 8. 2, 1, 9. Locus, 10. Patau's.

Q.184. What immediate assessment you will do in newborn?

Ans. Immediate assessment of newborn is completed by Apgar score. This score is developed by virginia Apgar in 1952. This score consist of observation of heart rate respiration muscle tone, reflex, irritability color of neonate. Each item is given score of 0–12 if criteria is strongly positive then it is 2 and if it is negative; then it is 0 (Zero). Normal score of baby is 8–9 if score is 5–7 it shows moderate difficulty of newborn to adjust to the extrauterine life if score is 4 or below 4 shows severe distress and may requires an endotracheal intubation.

- Short digits
- Single and palmar creases in hand
- Soft and short's hair
- Dry skin, septal defects

Small genitalia and infertility in males, duodenal atresia, oesophageal atresia, lymphoplastic leukemia can occur.

Q.181. What are the clinical manifestation of Klinefelter's syndrome.

Ans. These children present tall stature, poor musculature, small testis, delayed puberty, gynecomastia, infertile behaviour and emotional problems.

Q.182. Define genetic counseling.

Ans. According American Society of human Genetics "counseling is a communication process which deals with occurrence or risk of genetic disorder in family.

Q.183. Fill ups:

1. The portion of chromosome which codes for a character is called ________
2. Arrangement of chromosome in the cell is called ________
3. Trisomy 21 was first described by ________
4. The first famous clone born in ________ and named ________ (a sheep).
5. The ultra structure of chromosome is ________
6. The genetic make up of a person is called as ________
7. Down's syndrome is also known as ________
8. A male person affected with Klinefelter's syndrome have ________ X chromosome and ________ Y chromosome.
9. The position of gene on a chromosome is called ________
10. Trisomy 18 is also called as ________

Keys

1. Gene [illegible] Karyotype [illegible] Down [illegible] 1997 [illegible] 46 [illegible] Locus [illegible]
Edwards

Q.184. What immediate assessment you will do to newborn?

Ans. [illegible] assessment of newborn is conducted by Apgar score. This score is [illegible] and requires emergency medical attention.